D0629098

"*Daily PrayerWalk* is life changing. ⌐aying
that makes prayerwalking as natural as breathing and walking. I was
captivated by the illustrations of answered prayer and realized my own
prayer life will never be the same after reading this book."

—CAROL KENT, *president of Speak Up Speaker Services
and author of* Becoming a Woman of Influence

"*Daily PrayerWalk* is an insightful journey during which Janet inspires
us over and over that prayer makes a difference, and she offers great
practical advice to motivate us for a lifetime of both physical and spiritual health while influencing the lives of those around us."

—CHERI FULLER, *founder of Families Pray USA, speaker, and
author of* When Mothers Pray *and* When Couples Pray

"*Daily PrayerWalk* contains many good ideas for devotional prayer to
strengthen what prayerwalking has always been understood to be:
intercessory prayer on behalf of others, pursuing God's greater purposes in our communities."

—STEVE HAWTHORNE, *coauthor of* Prayerwalking: Praying On-
Site with Insight

"I've had the privilege of watching the transformation that prayerwalking can make in a life. *Daily PrayerWalk* takes us by the hand and
invites us to grow...to become all that God has created us to be...to
lay aside everything that so easily entangles us and run the race set

before us. Make 'prayerwalk' that race! Thank you, Janet, for a beautiful way to start each day."

—JOANNA WEAVER, *author of* Having a Mary Heart in a
Martha World

"*Daily PrayerWalk* will not only inspire you to listen to God's voice and to partner with him in ministry, but the fitness tips will motivate you to become physically fit as you walk and pray each day."

—CAROLE LEWIS, *First Place national director and author of*
Choosing to Change

"Friend to friend, Janet nudges me to lace up my walking shoes and follow my Savior into the new day. This is the camaraderie I have longed for: unguarded honesty from another follower and a new intimacy with the Lord."

—VIRELLE KIDDER, *conference speaker, radio host, and author*

Daily PrayerWalk

Meditations for a Deeper Prayer Life

Daily PrayerWalk

Janet Holm McHenry

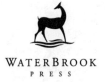

WATERBROOK
PRESS

DAILY PRAYERWALK

PUBLISHED BY WATERBROOK PRESS

2375 Telstar Drive, Suite 160

Colorado Springs, Colorado 80920

A division of Random House, Inc.

ISBN 1-57856-544-8

Published in association with the literary agency of Janet Kobobel Grant, Books & Such, 4788 Carissa Ave., Santa Rosa, CA 95405.

Library of Congress Cataloging-in-Publication Data
McHenry, Janet Holm.
    Daily prayerwalk : meditations for a deeper prayer life / Janet Holm McHenry.—1st ed.
        p.   cm.
Includes bibliographical references.
    ISBN 1-57856-544-8
    1. Prayer—Christianity—Meditations.   I. Title.
    BV210.3 .M34 2002
    248.3'2—dc21

                    2002003068

Printed in the United States of America
2002—First Edition

10 9 8 7 6 5 4 3 2 1

To my mother,
Doris Anne Fieg Holm,
who first taught me to pray

Contents

Acknowledgments

Writing a book about prayer is both a privilege and a responsibility, so I've needed many intercessors to pray for me. Many thanks to my prayer partners, One Heart writing sisters, and AWSA friends for keeping my hands held up.

I'm grateful for all those writers who've prayed and gone before me—those I've noted in this book and many more. I'm just a neophyte growing under your teaching.

I so appreciate the folks at WaterBrook Press, who have encouraged me in the writing of *PrayerWalk* and now this volume. Special thanks to Laura Barker, Michele Tennesen, Ginia Hairston, and Kirsten Blomquist. You mean a lot to me.

I can't say enough about Liz Heaney, my editor friend. She made me see clearly, work hard…and be a lot more sympathetic to my own students when I edit their papers. This book is graced with her gift.

Lastly, no book can be written without the support of one's family, and I lovingly thank my husband, Craig, and our children, Rebekah, Justin, Joshua, and Bethany, for letting me live out God's call.

To him be the glory.

God has changed my life through prayerwalking. He has also changed me over the last thirty years through a really great book—the Bible. As Christians we need both disciplines—daily prayer and daily study—in order to know God more intimately and to experience a deeper prayer life.

We're in training, you and I, and I'm excited about what God will do in both of us as we pursue our heart's desire to become more like Christ, our Personal Trainer in prayer and in life.

This book contains fifty meditations on prayer. Each one starts with a longer reading from the Bible called Daily PrayerWalk, as well as a PrayerWalk Focus—usually one verse—that you can use as a point of meditation as you start your prayer time, whether you walk or not. The text is a blend of teaching about the passage and others relating to the topic, as well as personal stories to help you see how God can work in our lives. Two other offerings follow each meditation: a Prayer Starter to help you pray about what you have read and a Fitness Tip for your walking regimen.

I pray you'll find great encouragement and help as you start your training, read God's Training Manual with me, and begin or continue your life of intercession.

I'll be praying for you!

Chapter 1

Why Pray?

PRAYERWALK FOCUS
Read Matthew 22:34-40.

DAILY PRAYERWALK
"Jesus replied: '"Love the Lord your God with all your heart and with all your soul and with all your mind."'"—Matthew 22:37

My friends are an important part of my life. I make conscious efforts to spend time with them—a day at a lake, an afternoon at a craft fair, a retreat weekend, dinner out. Through these and many other ways I've managed to stay in touch with high school friends, college roommates, and others, even with the demands of a full-time job and four children. I intentionally set aside time during the year to have face-to-face gatherings, with additional contact on the phone or through e-mail. I do this because I love my friends, they've been an important part of my life, and I enjoy spending time with them.[1]

I also feel that way about spending time in prayer with God, but this is a new attitude for me. Most of my Christian life I prayed because

I knew a good Christian should do such things. Other times I prayed when I was desperate—when life was falling apart and I couldn't juggle its demands or stresses anymore. Before I started prayerwalking, I'd been sensing that God wanted me to spend more time with him, to pray without my own agenda. I wasn't too sure what that all meant, and so I headed to the streets with my mental prayer lists for my family. As I was walking one morning, I saw a young father hand over his toddler girl to a day-care worker, and I was struck with the sense that God wanted me to pray for everything I saw as I walked.

Soon I began to sense God's presence as I prayed; in prayer I can partner with God. Now I pray for the same reasons I spend time with my friends: I love God, he is the most important thing in my life, and I enjoy spending time with him.

Jesus cares about why we pray. In the Sermon on the Mount, he told the crowd that blessed are the poor in spirit, those who mourn, those who are meek, those who hunger and thirst for righteousness, those who are merciful and pure in heart, those who are peacemakers, and those who are persecuted. If our prayers bring us closer to living out those characteristics, then we're praying for the right reasons.

Christ taught that more than anything God wants our hearts. He said, "'Love the Lord your God with all your heart and with all your soul and with all your mind.' This is the first and greatest commandment" (Matthew 22:37-38). We pray—and fast, read the Bible, give, worship—because we love God and wholly desire to develop lives that will glorify him.

I've thought a lot about why I pray and have put together this quiz for you and me:

I pray (check all that apply):
- ❏ to seek God's guidance
- ❏ for God's wisdom

- ❏ to feel closer to God
- ❏ to express my love for God
- ❏ to confess the junk of my life
- ❏ to escape the worries of the world
- ❏ to thank God for all he has given me
- ❏ to ask God to help me with my day
- ❏ to ask God to make me a better person
- ❏ to intercede for others
- ❏ because God wants me to spend time with him
- ❏ because God wants me to pray for others
- ❏ because I like talking with God
- ❏ because I know I should
- ❏ to impress other people
- ❏ other: _____

God is absolutely trustworthy.

When you have a friend like that, you certainly seek her out—call her on the phone for advice and regular chats, meet for lunch or a walk, go to a movie or shopping together. Similarly, my Lord has become my best friend, the one I can always depend on. Meeting with him each day, whether I'm prayerwalking or at home or in my car or in my classroom, is something I must do now—if only because being with Jesus has become my greatest joy.

PRAYER STARTER

Dear Lord, sometimes I pray only because I think it's expected of me. I want to make meeting you in prayer and in your Word the most important parts of my day—not to receive the approval of others but to simply learn more about the God I love. Help me to be more like your Son, who sought you continually for guidance, help, and companionship. In Jesus' name, amen.

FITNESS TIP

You may want to see your doctor before you start a walking routine if you check any of the following:

- ❑ My doctor has concerns about my cholesterol levels.
- ❑ I have a form of heart disease.
- ❑ I sometimes have pain in my chest or upper arms.
- ❑ I sometimes feel faint or dizzy.
- ❑ I haven't exercised in a year or more.
- ❑ My doctor says I need to lose weight.
- ❑ I have smoked in the last two years.
- ❑ I am taking a prescribed medication.
- ❑ Heart disease runs in my family.
- ❑ I have high blood sugar or diabetes.
- ❑ I have severe arthritis.
- ❑ I have chronic back or joint pain.
- ❑ I have recently had surgery or another medical problem that makes me physically weak.

Chapter 2

From the Inside Out

DAILY PRAYERWALK
Read Nehemiah 8.

PRAYERWALK FOCUS
"The joy of the LORD is your strength."—Nehemiah 8:10

As I have prayerwalked Main Street of my little town, I've witnessed a transformation of some of the homes and businesses. Our one and only gas station expanded into a minimart. The hardware store got a sandblasting and new varnish. The pharmacy is showing off a facelift—vinyl siding. I pray for the workers; I know it's not easy climbing up ladders and working in the elements.

I'm sure it wasn't easy for the Israelites, either, when they rebuilt the broken-down walls and burnt city gates of Jerusalem. When they were in captivity in Babylon, they had probably heard the passed-down stories of their beautiful promised city. But when they returned from captivity in Babylon—a century and a half after their ancestors were taken away—they found their fortified city in rock crumbles.

The vision of one man rebuilt the city walls: Nehemiah. His brother

Hanani had traveled the thousand-mile journey back to Babylon to tell him of the city's sad state. Within days of Nehemiah's arrival, the Israelites worked side by side to repair the wall. The third chapter of the book of Nehemiah lists all of the workers. The "next to him...beyond him...beside him...next to him" language makes me picture a Tom Sawyer row of workers, each setting rock and mortar into place. Less than two months after Nehemiah had arrived in Jerusalem, the Israelites had rebuilt the walls and gates, and the Jews' numerous enemies shrank away in fear, "because they realized that this work had been done with the help of our God" (Nehemiah 6:16). Party time—the people were ready to celebrate!

But even though the walls were rebuilt and the enemy had withered away, the people inside the city were still the same people—folks who were relying on the relationship their ancestors had had with God, not men and women who had their own relationship with him. But that soon changed.

At the party Ezra and the priests read from the Scriptures words that had never before pierced the hearts and souls of these people. They also prayed, and the hearts of the people began to change. In fact, their mourning and weeping from the reading of God's Word prompted this famous verse: "The joy of the LORD is your strength" (Nehemiah 8:10). They had thought that the walls of the city would be their strength; instead, they discovered that God's joy would be. When life presents stress, struggles, and even horror, the joy of knowing God can rise up within to give the believer the inner strength to keep going. For seven full days from sunrise to sunset, God's words penetrated their hearts, and the inside of Jerusalem—the people themselves—was changed as well.

Similarly, we can build a new physical exterior—we can exercise and work out—and still be a mess inside. I experienced this many years ago when I fanatically dieted and exercised and lifted weights and was down to a size six. But to do this I had substituted several compulsions for my overeating compulsion. My depression was probably the most severe during that time of my life. I expected life to be grand since my "shell" looked great, but I was just as empty as those Israelites behind their beautiful new wall.

Nehemiah and Ezra helped the Israelites discover the God of their ancestors by directing their prayers with praise. I have strengthened my "interior walls" because of the time I spend in praise when I prayer-walk. When I praise God, my focus moves from my needs and my concerns to God and his creation and his character. My self-orientation dissipates as I focus on his love and his provision for me. Before I began prayerwalking, I didn't pray much and I praised God even less. But when I began praying outside, in view of God's creation, praise came naturally.

The book of Nehemiah contains two kinds of praise. One simply recognizes who God is, as shown in "Blessed be your glorious name, and may it be exalted above all blessing and praise. You alone are the LORD" (Nehemiah 9:5-6). This form of high praise calls God by his different names, which are almost limitless. They include the Jewish words Jehovah, Elohim, El-Shaddai, and Adonai, and our limited translations I AM, Lord of Heaven, God Almighty, and Master.[2]

When I'm outside, I look up and see things everywhere that remind me of who God is. For example, if I see the stars dotting the early morning sky or the full, bright blue sky of midmorning, I praise my Creator. When I see the mountains still standing, I thank him for being my Sustainer. When two mountain peaks meet in a perfect V, I acknowledge God as the Architect. I think it's good to recognize these names for God, as they help to build my understanding of the One who has chosen me for eternity. There are days, though, when I find a name—a label of sorts—impossible for the One Who Caused All

Things into Existence. Ah, but now I've given him another name, haven't I?

The second form of praise in Nehemiah recognizes God for what he has done. "You made the heavens, even the highest heavens, and all their starry host, the earth and all that is on it, the seas and all that is in them. You give life to everything, and the multitudes of heaven worship you" (Nehemiah 9:6). God has done so much that we could fill our days listing all of his wondrous works.

When I start my day with praise, the problems that have troubled me don't seem as formidable. When I've remembered who God is and what he has done for me over the years, I know that I can trust him for my current struggles and concerns. Joy has replaced the depression that clouded my life for years. I think you'll find that as you praise him today, your walls will be rebuilt from the inside out as well.

Prayer Starter

Oh, Lord, my Lord, how majestic is your name in all the earth! When I consider the moon and the stars and all of creation, I know that your name is above all names. Let everything that lives and breathes bow down, for you alone are God. In Jesus' name, amen![3]

Fitness Tip

When you're just starting to walk, take it easy. Make a reasonable goal, considering your age and condition. You can always add on minutes, miles, and intensity! Don't exercise until you hurt—exercise as long as you feel good. Ten minutes is a reachable first-day goal. The next day add a few minutes. The following day try walking a little faster. *The 90-Day Fitness Walking Program* by Mark Fenton and Seth Bauer offers a day-by-day schedule to build a routine for someone who has struggled with fitness discipline.[4]

Chapter 3

Ordinary Faith, Extraordinary God

DAILY PRAYERWALK
Read Matthew 17:14-23 and 21:18-22.

PRAYERWALK FOCUS
"If you believe, you will receive whatever you ask for in prayer."
—Matthew 21:22

My faith is not extraordinary. I am just an ordinary woman who happens to know an extraordinary God. I know that the One who created the universe—the mountains that rise around my valley, the clouds that bring refreshment, the waning sun's rays that turn the skies into every color of red at sunset—is fully worthy of my trust and fully able to answer my prayer. My faith has grown as God has answered my prayers.

Jesus said, "If you have faith as small as a mustard seed, you can say to this mountain, 'Move from here to there' and it will move" (Matthew 17:20). We don't have to believe that the mountain will move; we just have to believe that God could move the mountain. That kind of faith requires that we recognize that the One who fashioned the peaks, geologic faults, volcanoes, and earthquakes could find the movement of a mountain a mere mustard-seed task.

Sometimes faith comes easily for me. For example, one before-dawn morning I watched a young, married man help his very expectant wife into their small pickup truck, and I prayed for their safe arrivals—couple and baby. A few days later I saw Mom carry the new bundle into their home for what I presumed was the first time. Simple requests like this don't require a stretch of faith, and they come and go easily in our prayer lives.

But what about those prayers of healing for a friend facing her sixth round of chemotherapy? How do we muster the faith to pray for something that doctors say won't happen? And if we don't have the faith that such a result would happen, should we even pray?

The disciples did not have this kind of faith at first. When Jesus healed a boy that they couldn't, they asked him why. He told them, "Because you have so little faith" (Matthew 17:20). He then added, "If you have faith…nothing will be impossible for you" (verse 20). When they wondered how his simple curse could wither a fig tree, Jesus said, "I tell you the truth, if you have faith and do not doubt, not only can you do what was done to the fig tree, but also you can say to this mountain, 'Go, throw yourself into the sea,' and it will be done. If you believe, you will receive whatever you ask for in prayer" (Matthew 21:21-22). Later God used the disciples to perform amazing miracles, so obviously their faith had grown.

How? Two faith-building miracles happened between Christ's teachings and the disciples' healings reported in Acts: the resurrection and the coming of the Holy Spirit, each promised by Christ. After these events the disciples became passionate leaders.

We are fortunate: We don't have to wait for a resurrection or the Holy Spirit. When I asked Christ into my life as a college sophomore, the Holy Spirit began living within me, and my walk of faith began. As I've sought out God's help through his Word and through prayer over the years, my prayers have become more faith-filled.

At the beginning of last year I started praying for a man I'd see early in the morning. I'd always prayed for safety on his job, but I started praying that he'd marry his "virtual" wife of twelve years or more. I was absolutely amazed just a few months later when I saw the announcement of their engagement in our little newspaper.

Another day I started praying for a young man that I'd often run across in the morning—that he'd come to know Christ in a personal relationship. Not long afterward I was again amazed to find my prayer in the process of being answered. The mother of a friend told me, "Pray for Todd. He has been coming to church every week and has been reading straight through the Bible."

What struck me most was the goodness of God in those answers. How could a couple who had been living together for years suddenly decide to get married? How could a sower of wild oats start going to church? Because of prayer? No! Because God is circumstantially—not coincidentally—working in the lives of people all around us. He invites us to pray with faith—not with something we muster with all our spiritual strength, but with the little seedlike faith that he has granted us and that can grow as we exercise it.

How do we pray in faith for our friend losing the battle to cancer? We pray to the God who resurrected his Son to heal our friend. We can pray that in full faith because we know that God has done and can do such a thing. Whether it's his will to do what we ask is another matter, though, so we don't have to be convinced that God will heal our friend in this life. We just have to be convinced that God *could* heal her. We only need to trust that he who allows crosses in our lives will redeem that pain with resurrection joy.

Join me with that little dot of faith and see what our extraordinary God will do in your community.

Prayer Starter

Dear Creator of heaven and earth, remind me continually "How great thou art." You are worthy of my faith-filled prayers. Thank you that I don't have to amass a mound of faith in scientific proportions that would tip the prayer scales in my behalf. You are trustworthy, and so I put my mustard-seed-sized faith in you and you alone. Grow me in my faith, Lord, through the reading of your Word and through a continual seeking of your presence in my life. In Jesus' name, amen.

Fitness Tip

If you want to invest in some workout clothes and your local stores don't carry an abundance, you can contact the following sources:

- RaceReady, 1-800-537-6868, www.raceready.com
- Road Runner Sports, 1-800-551-5558, www.roadrunnersports.com
- Title Nine (women's clothing only), 1-800-609-0092, www.title9sports.com

Chapter 4

God's Economy

DAILY PRAYERWALK
Read Matthew 19:16-30 (or Mark 10:17-31 or Luke 18:18-30).

PRAYERWALK FOCUS
"And everyone who has left houses or brothers or sisters or father or mother or children or fields for my sake will receive a hundred times as much and will inherit eternal life."—Matthew 19:29

People often ask me, "How do you get up that early to prayerwalk?" I still don't completely know. I could easily sleep longer every single morning, and at first getting up an hour earlier felt like a sacrifice, but now it's something I look forward to. I get less sleep now, but I've not had a cold or the flu during these three years of prayerwalking. I get less sleep, but somehow I'm healthier!

Saying yes to knowing God and following him means being willing to give up whatever it is that keeps us from him—an extra hour of sleep, a title, financial success, a paid-off mortgage. That's essentially what Jesus said to the rich, young ruler when he asked, "Teacher, what good thing must I do to get eternal life?" (Matthew 19:16). Jesus told him not only to obey the commandments, but also to give everything he had to the poor. The young man walked away dejected because he had great wealth.

If someone asked Jesus this question today, he might tell that person to give up his or her schedule. Time is a precious commodity to many of us. As a schoolteacher with a farmer husband, I'm not wealthy, but on many occasions I'd gladly give God my money rather than my time. I'd prefer donating dollars over making cookies for the youth group's bake sale. I'd rather give items to a charity auction than run the auction. For me, saying yes to Christ has meant giving him a full hour of my time every day just for prayer.

To do this I've had to give up some things that I enjoy doing: I don't go out regularly at night so that I can get to bed earlier. I don't watch television (we don't even have network television) and movies during the week. I don't allow even a good book (except the Bible) to tempt me beyond 9 P.M. But I have found those are small sacrifices for what I've received in return—greater intimacy with my Lord.

Scripture teaches that when we say yes to God, we gain so much more than we give up. When Peter asked Jesus what was ahead for his followers—"We have left everything to follow you! What then will there be for us?" (Matthew 19:27)—Jesus answered by telling his disciples that saying no to earthy things would mean a hundred times yes from God and eternal life (verse 29). Such a deal! Any stock market investor would jump at such dividends.

Recently I stood next to a man at the flagpole in front of the high school where I teach. We were holding hands with more than a dozen teens, and he was praying for them and our country in the aftermath of the attacks in New York City and Washington, D.C. I'd prayed for him over the last year as I walked past his home and heard him bellow at his family. Two months ago he committed his life to Christ and now plans to go into the ministry. Hearing this man pray reminded me yet again that the time I've invested in prayer has yielded great dividends—answers to prayers, improved physical and emotional health, and a more meaningful relationship with God.

Whenever we give up something in order to say yes to God, we'll always gain more than we give up—that's God's economy.

PRAYER STARTER

Dear Lord, thank you for sacrificing your all for me. Your coming to earth should have been enough for me to see how much you love me—but you died for me too. Help me remember how much you have given me and that what I return to you—my things, my gifts, my time—really is so little. I'll give you my all today, Lord! In Jesus' name, amen.

FITNESS TIP

Poor walking posture can lead to back and neck pain. When you walk, make sure your posture is correct. Casey Meyers offers the following head-to-toe checklist for good posture:

1. head straight (not tilted to either side) with chin parallel to the ground
2. shoulders level and loose, in line with the ears and directly over the hips
3. chest held moderately elevated, with the upper back erect
4. hips level and directly under the shoulders
5. knees and ankles straight and in line with hips, shoulders, and ears—back erect, chin parallel to the ground[5]

Chapter 5

On the Lookout

DAILY PRAYERWALK
Read 1 Peter 4:7-11.

PRAYERWALK FOCUS
"Watch unto prayer."—1 Peter 4:7, KJV

While on our way from northern California to the Los Angeles area to attend our daughter Rebekah's college graduation, we made a pit stop at a Taco Bell in the Stockton area. I was feeling cranky and stiff from sitting, but after I placed our order, I focused on the petite blonde who was stuffing our tacos into a plastic bag. I remembered that God had placed me there for a reason.

I wondered why this young girl was working at a Taco Bell during school hours. Had she dropped out of school? Could she have graduated the year before without skills for another kind of job? Did she also work at night to make ends meet?

Then I noticed that she was limping, so I asked, "Are you all right? Were you in an accident or something?"

She handed me the bag, looked into my eyes, and said, "My boyfriend hit me last night. He also jumped on me, and I'm not feeling so good." While I stood there, stunned, she hobbled over to get my drinks.

As she handed them over the counter, I told her, "Please get yourself out of that relationship. I'll be praying for you."

"Thank you," she said. "I hope I can."

I prayed for her for the rest of my trip. Every time I saw a Taco Bell, I asked God to remove her from that situation and redeem the pain of her life.

That morning—as I try to do every morning—I had asked God to help me be more observant of the people and circumstances around me so that I could intercede appropriately. I think that's what the apostle Peter meant when he wrote, "watch unto prayer" (1 Peter 4:7, KJV). I love this little phrase from the *King James*. Other versions offer their interpretation:

> "Therefore be clear minded and self-controlled so that you can pray." (NIV)

> "Therefore, be of sound judgment and sober spirit for the purpose of prayer." (NASB)

> "Stay wide-awake in prayer." (MSG)

Prayerwalking is careful, wide-awake, disciplined prayer.

Watch unto prayer. This one verse can be life changing. Imagine that God has you in each and every place and circumstance of your life for the purpose of prayer. Imagine that he wants you right where you are, to see and hear and sense the needs of folks around you—whether you're prayerwalking or not.

As you ask God to give you his eyes, you will begin to see prayer needs all around you. As you prayerwalk, you'll hear families argue. You'll hear curses uttered in frustration. As life becomes increasingly more threatening, you'll find more to pray about on behalf of those along your path. On the days I'm most aware of my purpose on earth, I'm praying all day long.

I don't think it's a coincidence when we become privy to other people's pain. Later on our trip Craig and I walked on Catalina Island off the coast of Los Angeles. There's a lovely promenade along the harbor of Avalon Bay that goes out to a point where a large round building, the Casino, houses a museum, ballroom, and theater. We passed a couple who had lingered after the movie showing had let out. They were arguing—she crying and accusing, he defending and apologizing.

As I heard the angry interchange, God reminded me that I was there on that island for more than just relaxation. I also was there to pray. So I prayed for them and then others we passed. I prayed for the shop owners who were still helping customers after 10 P.M., at the end of a thirteen-hour day. And I prayed for boat operators zipping here and there on busy Memorial Day waters.

Often I'll turn the wrong way or be delayed by traffic or find I've forgotten something and have to go back home to retrieve it. These circumstances used to frustrate me at my best, anger me at my worst. Now I see those occurrences as reasons to pray, obvious or not. Most of the time I'll never know the results of these prayers, but I believe God responds when his children watch and pray.

The next time you're standing in a long line at the bank or waiting in commuter traffic or growling because your spouse made the wrong turn, instead of getting impatient or frustrated, look for a reason to pray…and then do.

PRAYER STARTER

Father, make me ever watchful unto prayer today. Show me the needs of those around me as I walk and drive and work and play. Give me your eyesight so I will pray according to your will. In Jesus' name, amen.

FITNESS TIP

If you think others might not be able to notice you if you walk in the dark, you might want to buy sew-on or stick-on reflective patches—or even blinking lights—to attach to your clothing. Or consider getting some reflective paint that you can brush on your clothes, which will last through as many as fifty washes. A good investment is a reflective vest, about fourteen dollars. Sporting goods or discount stores carry these products.

Chapter 6

Removing Roadblocks

DAILY PRAYERWALK
Read Matthew 5:21-26.

PRAYERWALK FOCUS
"Therefore, if you are offering your gift at the altar and there remember that your brother has something against you, leave your gift there in front of the altar. First go and be reconciled to your brother; then come and offer your gift."—Matthew 5:23-24

Recently I found myself stuck in prayer. I was no longer sensing any communion or give-and-take with God. I'd pray, but he and I weren't exactly conversing. Then one morning Kent passed me in his car as I was prayerwalking, and I remembered that I hadn't resolved an issue at school with his son, Mike. Later that morning I asked Mike to stay after class a moment. I told him I had been wrong when I'd responded to him in sarcasm the week before and asked him to forgive me. He said, "Sure," and immediately I felt the roadblock between him and me lift. The next time I prayed I realized that the roadblock between God and me had been removed as well.

When I continually pray only to see no apparent answer to those prayers, I'm learning to look inward to see if I'm dirtied with unresolved sin. In Matthew 5:23-24 Christ teaches that if, when I'm making an offering to God, I remember that someone else is holding something against me, I'm to go and restore the relationship first, then make my offering. When we meet with God in prayer, I think we're making an offering of ourselves; we're giving our time and hearts and will. It's important to make sure things are right with others before we pray.

Does that mean that God hasn't forgiven me? No. Hebrews 10:10 teaches us that "we have been made holy through the sacrifice of the body of Jesus Christ once for all." It's a done deal with God, except for one thing—we still have to restore broken human relationships. Dag Hammarskjöld wrote of this need to be forgiven and to forgive:

> Forgiveness is the answer to the child's dream of a miracle by which what is broken is made whole again, what is soiled is again made clean. The dream explains why we need to be forgiven, and why we must forgive. In the presence of God, nothing stands between Him and us—we *are* forgiven. But we *cannot* feel His presence if anything is allowed to stand between ourselves and others.[6]

So while I look clean to God, my friend might still see the dirty mess who offended her. It's up to me to go to her and extend a sincere apology.

Along with essay writing and other skills, I often teach my students how to apologize and ask for forgiveness. Here's my formula:

I was wrong when I _____. Will you forgive me?

I tell them that a mumbled "sorry" isn't specific enough to acknowledge how we hurt someone and that if it seems insincere, the apology can add another layer of hurt. The words "I was wrong" show real repentance. When appropriate, we should also offer restitution. If you break your neighbor's lawn mower when you borrow it, you need to get it fixed or buy him a new one. If I make a mistake on a student's grade, I should apologize and adjust the grade. I can also call the parent right away or write a note so there's a clear understanding that the grade was my fault, not the student's.

I've found that when I use the above formula in a true spirit of caring, it usually touches the person and restores the relationship. Sometimes, though, the person decides to continue in anger and hurt. If I don't have peace about the situation, I'll continue to seek restoration. If I feel I've done what I can do, I just move on and trust that God will work things out.

Recently a friend said to me, "I need to know how to pray for someone who has hurt me deeply, who daily causes me pain." Sometimes we're the one who has been offended. If the offense turns to bitterness, then we become part of the roadblock even though we didn't initiate the offense. Jesus said, "When you stand praying, if you hold anything against anyone, forgive him, so that your Father in heaven may forgive you your sins" (Mark 11:25). We begin prayer with forgiveness. We forgive those who have hurt us so that when we confess our own wrongdoing, God will hear us and forgive us.

Is that easy? Nope! Forgiveness requires trust that God will take care of the other person, the whole situation, and me. Ultimately forgiveness is a huge step of faith that God is bigger than our personal baggage. Joseph forgave his brothers for conspiring to kill him, saying, "You intended to harm me, but God intended it for good to accomplish what is now being done, the saving of many lives" (Genesis 50:20). On the cross Jesus said, "Father, forgive them, for they do not know what they are doing" (Luke 23:34). If we model our prayer lives after Christ, we will not only seek forgiveness; we will also forgive.

PRAYER STARTER

Father, thank you for forgiving me. Remind me each day that I must be a peacemaker on your behalf. I want to seek others' forgiveness when I've hurt them and forgive those who've hurt me. Make me sensitive so that I'm aware when I tread on others' rights or feelings. In Jesus' name, amen.

FITNESS TIP

Here are some suggestions for how to remain motivated for a lifetime of walking:

- Set distance and intensity goals.
- Write down each day how far you go and your time.
- Find a partner who'll keep you accountable.
- Vary your route to add interest.
- Set up rewards for reaching a goal (food is probably not a good idea here).

Chapter 7

A Confident Approach

DAILY PRAYERWALK
Read Hebrews 4:14–5:10.

PRAYERWALK FOCUS
"Let us then approach the throne of grace with confidence, so that we may receive mercy and find grace to help us in our time of need."
—Hebrews 4:16

The principal of the school where I teach has an open-door policy for staff members, parents, and students. He welcomes visitors with a big smile, a bigger handshake, and the biggest hello you can imagine. His welcoming response always amazes me because I know he has a stack of demands on his desk. Even when his back is turned and he's at work at his computer, his door remains open just a few feet away from the busy hallway. All who enter are welcome and considered important, no matter who they are.

Scripture assures us that as Christians we have the same access to the Father—only more so. The writer of Hebrews tells us that we can "approach the throne of grace with confidence, so that we may receive mercy and find grace to help us in our time of need" (Hebrews 4:16). The reason we can turn to God with confidence—no matter how we are feeling or what we have done—is that we have a relationship with Jesus Christ, who is sitting at the right hand of the Father (Luke 22:69). Christ has bridged the gap between unholy us and our holy Father so that we may approach God confidently in prayer.

As our God-appointed advocate, Christ tells the Father, "Lord, don't look at Janet. Look at me. I died for this woman. She is not perfect, but I was the perfect sacrifice, and out of love I died for her. My death has already paid the penalty for anything she has done or will do."

No matter who we are, we can be confident that Christ welcomes us when we approach him in prayer. He hung out with those others would have spurned. For instance, he struck up a conversation with an adulterous Samaritan woman (John 4). He invited a tax collector named Matthew to be his disciple (Matthew 9:9-13). He allowed a prostitute to wipe his feet with her tears and perfume (Luke 7:36-50). Each one experienced the love of Christ, and when we pray, we feel his loving welcome as well.

According to Hebrews 7:25, Christ "always lives to intercede for [us]." The Greek word for *intercede* means "to plead for." As a go-between, Christ pleads with God for those things that are best for us. His words to the Father are perfect prayers.

This verse took on new meaning for me one morning recently when I didn't think God would want to listen to me. I didn't even want to get up. I'd worked late into the evening on schoolwork. I had a full day ahead at school and several extra hours afterward listening to senior project presentations. The dishes lay undone in the kitchen sink, and I was grouchy that no one else in the house had thought to help. *Why would God want to listen to me anyway?* I wondered. *I'm just going to spend the time complaining.*

Then I remembered Hebrews 7:25. Christ *lives* to intercede for us; it's the best part of his job, so to speak. Isn't that great? Even if I am grouchy and my prayers are a list of complaints, Christ can intercede and make them acceptable to the Father.

So I got up, confessed my pitiful state, and prayerwalked that morning, amazed at the thought that not only would Christ welcome grumpy me, but I would also give him pleasure by seeking his help through my prayers.

I love going places I know I'm welcomed, don't you?

PRAYER STARTER

Father, thank you for sending your Son who lives to advocate for me and to intercede on my behalf. When I'm not feeling worthy of entering your throne room in prayer, gently remind me that I may do so boldly because of the sacrifice your Son made for me. Allow him to deal gently with me, teaching me and showing me your ways. Thank you for such an empathizer, intercessor, and source of salvation. In Jesus' name, amen.

FITNESS TIP

One way to stay motivated to prayerwalk—or do any exercise—is to keep a diary or chart of your progress. Set specific distance and time goals. For example, you might decide that your goal would be to walk three miles in forty-five minutes. Give yourself three months or longer to meet the goal. Work up to the forty-five minutes first, then add intensity.

Chapter 8

Something Only God Can Do

DAILY PRAYERWALK
Read Luke 11:5-13.

PRAYERWALK FOCUS
"Ask and it will be given to you; seek and you will find; knock and the door will be opened to you. For everyone who asks receives; he who seeks finds; and to him who knocks, the door will be opened."—Luke 11:9-10

I've been known to overdo things for my kids. This is especially true on their birthdays. Craig and I don't give huge presents, but I do big parties. I try to create wonderful memories because I want my kids to know how special they are. Once I created a Wild West party for Joshua when he was in elementary school. The boys were cowboys; the girls, Indian princesses. We had target shooting and gold panning and lassoing. The kids munched my cowboy cake, served on blue enamelware, and used red bandanna handkerchiefs. We still talk about that birthday.

I love going nuts for my kids. I think God likes to go nuts for us too. After all, we're his kids. In Luke 11 Jesus asks, "Which of you fathers, if your son asks for a fish, will give him a snake instead? Or if he asks for an egg, will give him a scorpion?" (verses 11-12). Matthew recorded the following: "Which of you, if his son asks for bread, will give him a stone?" (7:9). Christ also teaches, "If you then, though you are evil, know how to give good gifts to your children, how much more will your Father in heaven give the Holy Spirit to those who ask him!" (Luke 11:13). God responds to our requests with loving generosity.

Here are a few more examples:

- He not only promised to rescue the Jews from slavery in Egypt, but also said he would lead them to a land *flowing* with milk and honey (Exodus 3:8).
- When the Shunammite woman asked for help to pay her debts, God provided enough oil not only to pay off her debts but also to live (2 Kings 4:1-7).
- When the Samaritan woman went to the well, she not only got a drink, but also received living water, eternal life, from Christ (John 4:13-14).

God gives to us abundantly when we boldly ask for something that's beyond our reach—something that only God can do.

I took God up on his offer when I began praying for my friend Rose. Originally a victim of breast cancer, she had been fighting bone cancer for nearly four years when Kim, another friend, heard about a facility in southern California operated by an oncologist who had an encouraging cure track record. She felt God directing her to raise thirty thousand dollars to send Rose immediately for the several-weeks-long procedures that would detoxify her body. We, Rose's friends, began to pray a bold prayer: that God would raise thirty thousand dollars in two weeks through the two thousand folks who live in our rural mountain area. And Kim began to knock on doors.

In less than two weeks we had raised more than forty thousand dollars. During that time another group of folks organized a dinner that raised over seven thousand dollars. Radio and television interviewers caught wind of the need and aired Rose's story. Children knocked on doors for aluminum cans. Eventually gifts of more than fifty thousand dollars were given to help Rose.

The generous response amazed all of us. It was far beyond what we expected. But God knew that the expenses would be greater than Kim had first estimated. He also knew the needs of others who are now benefiting from the funds raised in her name. We prayed and others prayed for a bold sum of money—and God overflowed our cups.

Now when I prayerwalk, I pray boldly.

PRAYER STARTER

Father, show me how to pray in a big way. Help me boldly ask you for those works that only you can do. Help my prayers extend beyond my reach, beyond my ability, even beyond my sight so that you alone are glorified. In Jesus' name, amen.

FITNESS TIP

Be a bold prayerwalker! Don't be afraid to walk when the weather is less than ideal. If you only walk when it's pleasantly warm outside, you'll probably miss half a year of walking. Take an umbrella when it rains. Put on boots when it snows. Walk before sunrise when it's hot. Consistency leads to discipline.

Chapter 9

Never Give Up

DAILY PRAYERWALK
Read Luke 18:1-8.

PRAYERWALK FOCUS
"Then Jesus told his disciples a parable to show them that they should always pray and not give up."—Luke 18:1

One of the schools my two oldest kids attended used to give character awards at the end of the year. For three years in a row Rebekah's principal handed her the Confidence Award—no surprise to Craig and me because of her outgoing nature. We had expected that she'd get the same honor her fourth and last year, but instead the Perseverance Award took its place next to the other three. The teachers were right: Rebekah has grown into a determined young woman who doesn't allow obstacles to stop her. Last spring she finished a five-year program in four years, because she had taken some of her required courses at three additional institutions when her own didn't offer the ones she needed at the right time. That's perseverance!

Jesus taught us to be persistent with our prayers. In Luke 18 he told the parable of the persistent widow. This woman would not give up! She had a legal case, and she was sure she was right. Day after day she'd knock on the judge's door, saying, "Grant me justice against my adversary" (Luke 18:3). Widows were especially vulnerable during Jesus' time. Without family or income, they could be taken advantage of. But not this woman—she was the squeaky wheel in that judge's courtroom.

One obstacle in her path was the judge himself. He didn't care about God or about people either. For quite some time, in fact, he tried to ignore this woman. But how do you ignore someone who keeps coming back into your courtroom, time after time? She kept making her argument with the judge over and over and over again until finally he said, "I will see that she gets justice, so that she won't eventually wear me out with her coming!" (Luke 18:5). Her perseverance convinced him that her point of view was correct.

Likewise, our persistence in prayer will have results as well. My friend Mary, a faithful prayerwalker, has been praying for her grand-daughter Christie for close to fifteen years. Beginning with her teen years, Christie made all the wrong choices. It almost seemed as though *no* were not in her vocabulary. Two babies arrived without a father. With drug addiction a constant companion, she kept losing jobs. Then she was arrested for stealing to support her habit. But one jail term didn't seem to make an impression. After she was released, Christie was back on drugs, pregnant for a third time, and eventually was put behind bars again.

When Christie was released from jail for the second time, Mary had her doubts that her granddaughter would finally get it together, but because she knew her Judge was good, she kept praying. Christie got a job and worked hard. Four years later she penned these words to her grandmother: "I love you and there were times in my life I couldn't remember where I lived that day, but I never forgot how much my grandma loved and prayed for me. That's the reason I'm not still a lost soul in the streets." Just as Jacob would not let go of the angel of God, Mary would not let go of a prayer stream for Christie.

This parable shows that even an unjust judge will grant a request when it's made day after day by a persistent petitioner. We're in a better position than the woman in the parable: Our Judge is good. Jesus said, "And will not God bring about justice for his chosen ones, who cry out to him day and night? Will he keep putting them off? I tell you, he will see that they get justice, and quickly" (verses 7-8). This Judge of ours wants us to persist with our prayers.

I will persist in prayer, week after week. Join me today and bring your petitions. Maybe we'll both someday receive the Perseverance Award.

PRAYER STARTER

Lord, I'm grateful that you are the Judge who hears my prayers. You even welcome the same ones over and over again. Day and night I will bring my requests to you, trusting that you know the perfect time for decision, the perfect way for the answer. In Jesus' name, amen!

FITNESS TIP

If you want your metabolism to kick up, try giving your walking workout a boost. After a warmup, on a straight road lined with utility poles (usually one-tenth of a mile apart), walk at a rapid pace for two or more poles, then walk more moderately for the same distance. Repeat this pattern, remembering to cool down slowly at the end.

Chapter 10

Keep It Simple

Read Matthew 6:7-13.

PRAYERWALK FOCUS

Our Father which art in heaven,
Hallowed be thy name.
Thy kingdom come.
Thy will be done in earth, as it is in heaven.
Give us this day our daily bread.
And forgive us our debts, as we forgive our debtors.
And lead us not into temptation, but deliver us from evil:
For thine is the kingdom, and the power, and the glory, for
ever.
Amen. (Matthew 6:9-13, KJV)

If you asked my husband if I am a woman of many words, he'd probably think of my fifth appendage—the phone—and say yes. I was, however, trained as a journalist in the days when journalistic writing was spare. *Who, what, when, where, why,* and sometimes *how* filled up a dozen or so inches of newspaper copy, enough for what the reader usually needed to know.

But we don't need to use a lot of words in order to pray effectively. In fact, Jesus used a simple prayer as an example of how we should pray. In the Lord's Prayer Jesus models efficiency in prayer. With just a few clauses, he teaches us how to offer praise, to pray for God's will, to ask for our basic needs, and to request forgiveness and protection. That's a lot in a nutshell!

Apparently we don't need fancy words or elaborately reasoned explanations to make our point with the Father. But this can be hard for someone like me. As an English teacher, I'm tempted to pray in traditional essay form: tell God what I'm going to say, say it, then tell him what I've said. But I don't need to give God five long paragraphs about why my ten-year-old car should be replaced; I can just ask for his provision for something more reliable. He knows the long list of reasons. I think he'd rather know that I trust him for everything I need. It's not wrong to elaborate or pray at length; it's just that we don't have to. It's okay to keep our prayers simple in nature—minus the rationale, minus the flowery word choice, minus the padding.

Right before he gave the disciples this example of how to pray, Jesus said that some people prayed empty words over and over in the hopes that their many words would gain an answer (verse 7). According to one commentary this is like praying according to the "slot-machine" principle—if I put enough quarters in and pull the handle enough times, then I'll win a favorable response from God.[7] But God doesn't need to hear a lot of words. He wants our sincere hearts that trust in his goodness.

Recently my son Justin called from school. He needed money, he said. His car insurance was due. He had to pay his registration. Getting out of a bad apartment situation had taken all his food money. He'd run out of Top Ramen. Sure I cared about all the details, but I'd already started for the checkbook when he said "insurance." I know my kids only ask for money when they really need something. And I'll help as much as I'm able. After all, I love them! How much more true is that for our heavenly Father—but he has no limits on what he is able to give.

So when I'm prayerwalking, I like to keep my prayers to the point. I ask for protection for commuters. I ask for a blessing for the business owners. If I know of a personal need in the family, I ask God to intervene, all the while praying that these folks will grow in their relationship with God. What I've found, frankly, is that there are just so many needs in my community I can't elaborate—and often I don't know the details anyway. That doesn't mean I don't care; I know that God doesn't need a full discourse on each situation. "God is in heaven and you are on earth, so let your words be few" (Ecclesiastes 5:2). We can keep it simple. God knows all the details.

PRAYER STARTER

Father, I praise you, for you are my holy God. May your will be done in my life and in my community. Thank you for your continued provision for my family and me. Forgive me for those times when I haven't done your will, Lord—and keep me mindful to forgive others their failures too. Protect me, Father, and keep me in your care. In Jesus' name, amen.

FITNESS TIP

On days when you're facing a time crunch, simplify your routine. Go for a shorter walk, even just ten minutes. God knows when you have a full day. It's better to meet him for just those ten minutes than to miss entirely. Besides, it's always harder to get motivated after skipping a day—for whatever reason.

Chapter 11

Help!

Read Numbers 11:4-25.

PRAYERWALK FOCUS
"I cannot carry all these people by myself; the burden is too heavy for me."—Numbers 11:14

Here's a trivia question: What's the shortest prayer? I'm guessing it's "Help!" This may be the most common prayer as well. When life gets overwhelming, many of us cry "Help!" in our prayers.

I prayed this simple prayer one day last spring. I had been working late hours at the high school, signing students up for next year's classes, tutoring, and supervising senior project presentations. My piles of essays were growing. I was helping my daughter with wedding plans, doing radio interviews in the cracks of my schedule, and writing and speaking on weekends. Dinners had almost become nonexistent at our house. In fact, I had gotten so busy that I'd started using a trick I learned from the teenagers I teach—writing my lists on my left hand, since I couldn't even remember where my lists were. Then a week before school ended, I forgot about an interview, missed a dental appointment, and nearly got my students' grades in late. All in one day!

"Help!" I prayed the next morning.

Many people throughout the Bible called out to God for help, including Moses, who was leading a couple of million Jews out of captivity in Egypt. In Numbers 11 the Israelites had grown sick of only having God's miracle manna to eat. They wanted the fish, cucumbers, melons, leeks, onions, and garlic they remembered from Egypt and complained—loudly! Verse 10 says Moses heard *every family* wailing outside their tents about the food, and we know from Exodus 12:37 that this could mean as many as 600,000 families. I don't know about you, but when just *my* five family members complain about what I've fixed for dinner, that's more wailing than I want to hear!

Moses does a little wailing of his own. I don't consider this a minor wail either: He rants at God:

> Why have you brought this trouble on your servant? What have I done to displease you that you put the burden of all these people on me? Did I conceive all these people? Did I give them birth? Why do you tell me to carry them in my arms, as a nurse carries an infant, to the land you promised on oath to their forefathers? Where can I get meat for all these people? They keep wailing to me, "Give us meat to eat!" I cannot carry all these people by myself; the burden is too heavy for me. (Numbers 11:11-14)

He even asks God to allow him to die rather than face the continued burden of the Jews' complaining. Moses' prayer could be summed up in one word: "Help!" He recognized that he couldn't do it all by himself anymore.

God's answer was simple and immediate. He instructed Moses to appoint seventy elders, and then God put the Spirit on them. God didn't remove Moses from the situation, instead he lightened Moses' burden by giving him helpers.

When I yelled "Help!" God answered me right away too. A schedule change at school gave me a full day without students to get caught up on my paperwork. One of my teacher's assistants took over textbook collection without my asking and did a better job than I usually do. The radio interview load lightened until school ended for the summer, and I decided to take a few months' leave from teaching a class at church. I even made it through the school year without having to write any more lists on my left hand.

I am learning to ask God to help me through all the crazy events of my day *before* it even begins, before I am desperately trying to juggle and struggle to remember every last detail of a mental list. I want to know at the end of the day that I've been aware of God's presence and all I did that day was good in his eyes. So I whisper, *"Help."* Who better to consult than the One who told Moses, "Is the LORD's arm too short?" (verse 23)?

PRAYER STARTER

I'm sorry, God, that sometimes I forget to take my daily to-do lists to you—my work schedule, my errands, the demands others are making of me. Help me start each new day with a simple word: *help.* I want to be desperate for your caring touch. Let me feel this desperateness when I forget to turn over these simple wants and needs and concerns. Guide me clearly in your will. In Jesus' name, amen.

FITNESS TIP

If you want to be an aggressive aerobic walker and are overweight or have a history of heart problems, you might want to invest in a heart-rate monitor (please check with your doctor). The monitors are available at good sports-equipment stores or through Creative Health Products, Inc., 1-800-742-4478.[8]

Chapter 12

Praying the Bible

DAILY PRAYERWALK
Read Psalm 119:1-48.

PRAYERWALK FOCUS
"Blessed are they whose ways are blameless, who walk according to the law of the LORD."—Psalm 119:1

At times we just don't know how to pray.

The situation may just be so hard that words fail us. That was true for many of us after the attacks on the World Trade Center and the Pentagon; we had no words to express our horror and grief. Instead of just staring blankly during times like this, I've found it helps to turn to the Bible to guide my prayers. The psalms have become a refuge for me, particularly the laments on those days when life has seemed so overwhelming. In the months since the attack on our country, I've been praying that God will be our refuge, shield, and stronghold (Psalm 18:1-2).

I also pray the Bible when I want to pray for God's will. A writer friend of mine has a son who struggled for years with alcohol and drug addictions. We prayed and prayed for him. He'd make a commitment to change, then fall back into the same habits. Daily she'd entrust her child to God and nearly daily find her son desperate again—and she'd be ashamed at times to report to her praying friends how he'd failed once more. Wasn't it God's will that her son be released from the claws of drugs and alcohol?

One night as I searched the Bible for guidance, I noticed this verse: "Yet I am not ashamed, because I know whom I have believed, and am convinced that he is able to guard what I have entrusted to him for that day" (2 Timothy 1:12). I shared that verse with my friend and began praying it for her son. A short time later he entered a Christian rehabilitation facility. He has now been clean for many months and is witnessing to others in his family of God's faithfulness.

Praying the words of Scripture can also give life to my prayers when my own words seem stale. This past year held a couple of significant milestones for my daughter Rebekah. Not only did she graduate from college, but five weeks later she married her best friend, Ozzie. For weeks before the wedding I prayed for an apartment for them. They had looked for a place near her future job and his college campus but hadn't found anything they could afford.

One day I came across this verse in the Bible: "Even the sparrow has found a home, and the swallow a nest for herself…a place near your altar, O LORD Almighty, my King and my God" (Psalm 84:3). I began to pray that God, who finds even birds a nest, would provide a home for Rebekah and Ozzie—even near their church. On Rebekah's college graduation day I asked if they had inquired at the apartment building where she was living. The story is short. They hadn't. They did. They signed.

So how do I pray the Bible? I simply read the verses, think about how God's words could become my own, and then reword the scripture as a prayer. Here's how I would make Psalm 119:1-7 my own prayer—no fancy words, no editing:

Lord, I want to obey you, so that I might be found blame-
  less.
Bless me when I am seeking you with all of my heart.
Help me make no mistakes, and teach me to walk in your
  ways.
You have given us words that are to be fully obeyed.
I pray that I can follow your words diligently.
I don't want to cause you shame by slipping.
Instead, I will praise you with an upright heart
As I learn more about your Word each day.
Don't forsake me, Lord—
I promise to obey your laws.

When the words of the Bible sincerely become our own, we get to know God more fully and allow the Truth to change our hearts.

Before you prayerwalk, do a little walking through the Word and allow it to become your prayer focus.

PRAYER STARTER

Lord, help me keep my way pure by living according to your Word. I will seek you with all of my heart; please help me not stray from your commands. I am putting your Word into my heart so that I will not sin against you. I praise you with my lips and rejoice as I read about the life you have given me. In Jesus' name, amen.[9]

FITNESS TIP

If you prefer the idea of walking to get somewhere, consider these goal-oriented walks: to work, to the store, to the park, to a friend's house, to your kids' school. Either walk the return trip, or arrange for someone on the other end to give you a ride home.

Chapter 13

Pulling Rank

DAILY PRAYERWALK
Read John 14:1-14.

PRAYERWALK FOCUS
"I will do whatever you ask in my name, so that the Son may bring glory to the Father."—John 14:13

Growing up I believed that I was the most important little girl in the whole world. After all, I was Bob Holm's daughter. My father was assistant manager of Marsh's Department Store in Hudson, New York, and he ran the entire building, or so it seemed to me. I could whoosh through the revolving front doors of that multistoried brick building on Warren Street, and I was special. The ladies in cosmetics and jewelry and the men's department would warmly greet me and rush around to find out where my father was.

Dad was never too busy to give me a hug and ten cents. With dime in hand, I'd go into the employees' lunchroom, pick out a bottle of Coca-Cola and a candy bar, and leave my dime in the dish. No one questioned me when I would stay there and finish my prizes. I could have asked for almost anything, and anyone in the building would have done it. I was the little princess of Marsh's Department Store—all because my daddy was the king.

We have the same privileged position as children of the King of kings. We aren't put on hold because of call waiting or forced to listen first to a dozen recorded messages. We've got a hotline to the Father! We know him personally!

Three times we read in John:

"And I will do whatever you ask in my name, so that the Son may bring glory to the Father. You may ask me for anything in my name, and I will do it." (John 14:13-14)

"Then the Father will give you whatever you ask in my name." (John 15:16)

"I tell you the truth, my Father will give you whatever you ask in my name." (John 16:23)

What does it mean to pray in Jesus' name? It's more than just saying "in Jesus' name" at the end of a prayer. This means that our prayers should bring glory to God (John 14:13) and actually carry on Christ's work (John 14:14). It's more than imagining "WWJP" (What Would Jesus Pray?). It's also seeing what Jesus is now doing in my life…and perhaps someone else's life…and praying according to the work I see God doing.

In biblical times a person's name signified who he was. If I use Christ's name in prayer, my prayers should bring credit to him, not any disrepute. Even the use of his name is done prayerfully.

After my sophomore year in college I worked in Washington, D.C., at the Posthumous Division of the Awards Branch of the Department of the Army. There I answered correspondence from families inquiring about their children's awards from the Vietnam War. On my stacks were letters forwarded from the offices of U.S. senators and congressmen and the president. Those letters were given priority because the addressee had sent them through those advocates. In the same way, when Jesus asks us to pray in his name, he's asking us to pray prayers that would be worthy of his name.

Every time we whoosh through heaven's doors with another request of the Father "in Jesus' name," we can be recognized as a princess or prince and get immediate hearing because we know Jesus Christ personally.

The privilege of knowing Christ and using his name bears with it the responsibility of living up to that name. Just because I was Bob Holm's daughter didn't mean I could get away with running through the store, messing up merchandise, and snitching a lollipop from the candy counter. What I did reflected on my father.

The same is true for us.

PRAYER STARTER

Dear heavenly Father, thank you for the privilege of knowing you through your Son, Jesus Christ. May I never abuse the privilege of our relationship but only come to you with a sincere and humble heart in prayer. Show me how I can share this intimate privilege with others so that they, too, can experience the joy of using your Son's name. In Jesus' name, amen.

FITNESS TIP

Your feet shouldn't blister if your shoes fit well. Here are some precautionary measures you can take to avoid blisters if you plan an extra long walk:

- Rub petroleum jelly on your toes.
- Powder them to cut down on friction.
- Wear extra socks.

If they hurt afterward, try massaging them with a minted foot cream.

Chapter 14

Faith-Building Signs

Read Isaiah 7:1-25.

PRAYERWALK FOCUS

"Again the LORD spoke to Ahaz, 'Ask the LORD your God for a sign, whether in the deepest depths or in the highest heights.'"—Isaiah 7:10-11

When we're praying for something over the long haul—years for a prodigal child or a nonbelieving spouse, for example—sometimes we just need a little piece of encouragement from the Lord so that we don't lose heart. As I've prayed for my son through this valley time of his commitment, God has graciously given me signs that Justin will return to him.

The strongest of these signs has been in the form of poetic words. The first was the poem "Standing in the Gap" by Shirley Pope Waite that I found in my devotional Bible.[10] Her five stanzas proclaim that she'll stand in the gap of prayer every day until her son reclaims the faith of his youth. The poem has been such a strong sign of hope to me that I think I've about got it memorized. Over the years I've also shared it with other moms who have struggled in prayer over their sons. It has helped me hope that my son will reclaim the faith he proclaimed as a boy and has encouraged me to keep standing in the prayer gap for him.

I've not been alone in asking God for a sign; several biblical characters did as well—and God honored those requests. When Abraham sent his servant to a distant land to find a bride for his son Isaac, the servant prayed that he'd meet such a girl at the town well—that she'd even offer to draw his water (Genesis 24). It's the longest engagement story in the Bible, but God honored the servant's request for such a sign. In this case God gave the sign for clarity so that a simple servant could know without a doubt that Rebekah was the right bride for Isaac.

When the Jews needed a warrior judge, God appointed Gideon (Judges 6). But Gideon, the youngest of the weakest clan, was unsure that he could rally the Jews against the Eastern peoples who had invaded the Jews' land. First, he asked for a sign that it was really God talking to him, so God consumed Gideon's offering with instant fire that arose out of the rock. Later when the massive armies of opposition crossed the Jordan, Gideon asked for two more signs that God would save Israel through Gideon. Test one: God put dew on the wool fleece but not on the ground. Test two: God made the fleece dry when the ground was wet. Those signs assured Gideon that God would help him save Israel. Gideon went on to defeat the invaders with a small fraction of his army's original size.

God even invited King Ahaz to ask for a sign. Two countries were trying to get Judah's king, Ahaz, to join forces with them against Assyria. Ahaz was considering joining Assyria against them. But God wanted his people to trust him for protection, not to make pacts with countries like Assyria that did not acknowledge him. So he told Ahaz, "Ask the LORD your God for a sign, whether in the deepest depths or in the highest heights" (Isaiah 7:11).

In this case God offered a miracle sign to bring about the faith of a man who had not acknowledged God, who had even sacrificed to other gods. But Ahaz refused the offer. God was willing to help grow Ahaz's faith, but Ahaz would not give the Lord the chance. Assyria temporarily helped out Judah but eventually devastated it.

God chose to give the sign anyway. It was promised through Isaiah's prophecy: "The virgin will be with child and will give birth to a son, and will call him Immanuel" (Isaiah 7:14). The fulfillment of that sign came with the birth of Christ. The sign gave promise not only to Jews, but also to all the earth, that God cared enough about us to come to earth to demonstrate his sacrificial love.

While these examples demonstrate that it's okay to rely on signs once in a while, we shouldn't get into the habit of asking for them. If we expect God to always give us a sign, it's akin to asking him to prove himself—and we will live out our lives lacking true faith. Jesus told Satan—after he had tempted Jesus a for a third time to doubt God— "Do not put the Lord your God to the test" (Luke 4:12). If we're always asking for signs, we've lost sight of what the word *faith* means— "being sure of what we hope for and certain of what we do not see" (Hebrews 11:1).

But when we need encouragement from God—that he cares about our prayers for our family and community—we can expect that he will bless us with a gift of hope. He did this for me again just recently through another poem, "Prodigal," written by T. L. Marshall in *Decision* magazine.[11] The prodigal son tells of his long trip back home to his father, who greets him warmly. That poem gives me hope that eventually my son, too, will understand that the longings of his heart will only be met as he returns home to his heavenly Father. It has also reminded me that the Father longs for my son's return as much as I do.

PRAYER STARTER

Lord, thank you for the lengths to which you have gone to help build my faith. Thank you that your story is written down so my trust of you can grow day by day, simply by reading your Word. Help me to be expectant as I pray but not expect that you have to prove yourself to me. In Jesus' name, amen.

FITNESS TIP

To figure your aerobic target zone, follow these steps:
1. Subtract your age from 220.
2. Multiply this number by .5.
3. Also multiply the number from number 1 above by .75.

The numbers you get in 2 and 3 above will give you your aerobic target range. My aerobic target range is between 85 and 128 heartbeats per minute. Less than 85 beats would probably not be considered aerobic; more than 128 may be dangerous. Verify your target range with your doctor.

Chapter 15

A Thankful Heart

DAILY PRAYERWALK
Read Psalm 107.

PRAYERWALK FOCUS
"Give thanks to the LORD, for he is good; his love endures forever."
—Psalm 107:1

When I pray, I usually begin with praise and thanksgiving. Praise recognizes who God is; thanksgiving recognizes what God has done. Praise acknowledges God himself; thanksgiving acknowledges his actions. I don't worry about keeping the two separate—God knows which is which! While I'm not an advocate of praying by formula—prayer should be a natural discourse with God—I do like to begin my prayers by focusing on what I'm grateful for. It just seems right to thank God for what he has done before I ask for something more!

When we give thanks in prayer, we are recognizing the work of God, from the simple to the miraculous. The biblical writers often did this. In most of his letters Paul tells the church or individuals how he gives thanks to God for them; he told the Thessalonians that he thanked God for their faithful and love-filled work and their hope-inspired endurance (1 Thessalonians 1:3). Solomon thanked God for the opportunity to fulfill his father's desire for a temple (1 Kings 8:15). Daniel thanked God for telling him what the king's dream meant (Daniel 2:19-23). Jesus also gave thanks, including a thanksgiving for the five loaves and two fish that he distributed to five thousand, with twelve baskets left over (John 6:11).

The challenge comes when we're reminded to "give thanks in *all* circumstances, for this is God's will for you in Christ Jesus" (1 Thessalonians 5:18, emphasis added). How do you do that through a divorce? The loss of a home to fire? The death of someone you love, especially in unfair circumstances? I'm not going to make light of any of those situations. This has got to be one of the hardest things we're asked to do as Christians—to give thanks in the awful situations of our lives.

It doesn't make sense. But that's the nature of the gospel: It doesn't make sense. It's paradoxical that Christ would give life through his death. That when others are despairing, believers have hope. That when facing death, believers have peace. Faith implies a leap. It doesn't make sense. But awful things will happen even to those who believe; it may be our thankful response that helps someone else take that leap of faith. Giving thanks in *all* circumstances, even bad ones, is a small, trustful step—that God will take the pain, make us more like Christ because of it, and perhaps even redeem it in ways we could not even anticipate. The spiritual strength to take this step comes from God—as we pray, read his Bible, and choose to trust—even when it doesn't make sense.

If you are a novice at thanking God, you might use Psalm 107 as a model. The psalm is believed to have been written by a Levite (one of the priestly clan) for use in worship at an annual festival. It begins:

Give thanks to the LORD, for he is good;
his love endures forever.
Let the redeemed of the LORD say this—
those he redeemed from the hand of the foe,
those he gathered from the lands,
from east and west, from north and south. (verses 1-3)

The psalm reminds us to thank God for saving us, for pursuing us, for dying for us. The rest of the psalm lists what God did to take care of the Israelites. He fed them in the desert. He led them to just the right place. He saved them when they returned to him. He stilled storms and turned deserts into pools of water and blessed their harvests. The psalm recounts a long history of the Lord's involvement with his people. We don't have to recount our history with God every time we pray, but this is just an example of the kinds of things we can remember in our prayers of appreciation.

Whether we're in our prayer closet at home or on the streets prayer-walking, we can thank God for the simple instances of his care. For preventing that car accident. For giving us wisdom about how to discipline our child. For teaching us to bite our tongues when our first instinct would be to lash out. For helping us see our pride and giving us a repentant heart. For saving our town from flood or fire or drought. For helping us give thanks in all circumstances, even ones that are hard.

PRAYER STARTER

Dear Father, create in me a thankful heart, one that takes long enough to pause and reflect over the good things—and even hard circumstances—that you've brought or allowed in my life. Help me be observant and recognize your hand and then to take the time to be thankful to you as I walk throughout my day. In Jesus' name, amen.

FITNESS TIP

If you're walking to encourage weight loss, it's important to be careful about what you eat. Sometimes there's a tendency to eat more because you figure, "Oh, well, I'm exercising every day!" It's possible to walk every day and even gain weight if you're not watchful of your food intake.

Chapter 16

Heartfelt Confession

DAILY PRAYERWALK
Read Psalm 51.

PRAYERWALK FOCUS
"Create in me a clean heart, O God; and renew a right spirit within me."—Psalm 51:10, KJV

If the proverbial umbilical cord hasn't snapped by the time you and your child begin planning a wedding, that's the time it'll happen. Rebekah and I certainly found that planning a wedding five hundred miles apart is a bit challenging, especially since we often had very different ideas about what was appropriate. I blew it a lot. I thought I knew the right place and the right kind of invitations and even the right folks for the wedding party. I'd forgotten that it wasn't my wedding. It was Bekah and Ozzie's. I had to ask my daughter's forgiveness several times for getting pushy, getting angry, and getting uptight about money.

King David blew it big time too. Because he was attracted to Uriah's wife, Bathsheba, and had gotten her pregnant, David had Uriah sent to the battlefront, where he would certainly be killed. He was, and

David married Bathsheba, probably thinking no one would know his dirty deed. But God knew and reprimanded David through the prophet Nathan:

> Why did you despise the word of the LORD by doing what is evil in his eyes? You struck down Uriah the Hittite with the sword and took his wife to be your own. You killed him with the sword of the Ammonites. Now, therefore, the sword will never depart from your house, because you despised me and took the wife of Uriah the Hittite to be your own. (2 Samuel 12:9-10)

We don't see David praying when he was lusting after a woman who was not his wife or when he had her brought to him or when he found out she was pregnant or even after Uriah was killed in battle. We don't see David praying at all until Nathan confronted him with God's displeasure.

Much pain certainly resulted from David's sin—not only Uriah's death and Bathsheba's grief, but also the death of the child born of David and Bathsheba's adulterous union. However, one good thing—Psalm 51—resulted from David's eventual repentance: "I have sinned against the LORD" (2 Samuel 12:13). It's the classic penitential prayer. In the psalm David made it clear how he intended to follow through with his repentance and how he hoped God would help him.

• He recognized his sin and its effect.

> Have mercy on me, O God…
>> blot out my transgressions.
> Wash away all my iniquity
>> and cleanse me from my sin.
>
> For I know my transgressions,
>> and my sin is always before me. (verses 1-3)

- He asked God to forgive him and cleanse his heart.

  Cleanse me with hyssop, and I will be clean;
      wash me, and I will be whiter than snow. (verse 7)

- He asked God to restore him.

  Let me hear joy and gladness;
      let the bones you have crushed rejoice.
  Hide your face from my sins
      and blot out all my iniquity.

  Create in me a pure heart, O God,
      and renew a steadfast spirit within me.
  Do not cast me from your presence
      or take your Holy Spirit from me.
  Restore to me the joy of your salvation
      and grant me a willing spirit, to sustain me.
          (verses 8-12)

Likewise, in our prayers of confession we need to take responsibility for our sin, seek a restored relationship with the Father, and be willing to make significant changes in our lives.

True confession implies that we are not only sorry, but that we've also turned completely away from that sin and have done something concrete to rectify the results that our wrongdoing may have caused. If we're staying close to the Lord in prayer, we know that the Holy Spirit will convict us of our offenses and not let us walk any further until we've restored our relationship with him and those we've hurt.

I'm grateful that God convicted me of my need to ask for Rebekah's forgiveness. As a result the bigger wedding picture turned out great—all 150 of them! And what amazed me the most was not how beautiful Rebekah looked (she's always gorgeous), but how happy I looked. We had put behind us all the difficult phone calls and long debates, our relationship was restored, and, even better, it was the most fun wedding I've ever attended. How many mothers of the bride can say that?

PRAYER STARTER

Father, create a pure heart within me. Keep me so close to you that the instant I sin, I'm stung by the separation's pain. Thank you that I am washed with the blood of Jesus so I can confess and be restored into joyful fellowship with you. In Jesus' name, amen.

FITNESS TIP

You can buy hand weights that fill with water to adjust the weight. Put more water in before you start as you're ready for a more challenging workout. They can also be used as water bottles, too. As you begin to feel fatigued, pour out or drink the water.

Chapter 17

Prayer Gossip

DAILY PRAYERWALK
Read Proverbs 11:12-25.

PRAYERWALK FOCUS
"A gossip betrays a confidence, but a trustworthy man keeps a secret."—Proverbs 11:13

Many years ago I received a prayer request for a teenage girl who had filed rape charges against a teenage boy. Both had been my students, and I passed the prayer request along and along and along. The girl eventually dropped the charges, but some young people became upset with me, as they figured out I'd cast my judgment on the boy and prejudiced others' viewpoints as well. That incident taught me that we do not need to spread other people's personal lives all over the community.

Anytime I tell others something that could perceivably hurt someone's reputation, I am gossiping—even when my words are couched as a prayer request. In Proverbs we learn that "A gossip betrays a confidence, but a trustworthy man keeps a secret" (11:13). In other words, when someone tells us something in confidence, we should keep the information to ourselves. A few words—despite their truth—can ruin a person's reputation and break up relationships.

We gossip when we give a prayer request and even when we pray aloud, particularly if we reveal something that had been given in confidence. Here are some examples of what I call "prayer gossip":

"Please pray for Jessica. She told me that she is having an affair."

"Harry needs prayer so he can stop gambling online."

"Father, I'm really worried about Billie. I think she has an eating disorder."

Our words about others usually do one of two things—build them up or tear them down. When I reveal deeply personal and private information about someone else's struggles and sins, I am out of line unless I have that person's permission to do so.

I've experienced firsthand the hurt that "prayer gossip" can cause. When I asked for prayer for one of my children, I trusted a friend to keep the details to herself. She did not, and word got back to me that another friend had expressed a very unkind comment about my child. Oh, that hurts when you're already in pain.

If I spread prayer gossip about someone, what I may be doing is holding myself up as better than that other person. Jesus tells us to do the opposite—to humble ourselves (Luke 18:14). When we pray humbly, we truly seek someone's good. That can be done even with public prayer—even frequent intercession on someone's behalf—when it's done in a manner that lends dignity to the individual, not embarrassment.

The Internet has become a great way to share prayer requests, and I use it to exchange them with my friends. But I don't have to provide all the gory details. "Please pray for my friend in Kansas who has breast cancer" is enough. Dozens have prayed for "Janet's friend with breast cancer." One woman I've not even met even sent me a book to send to her. Isn't that neat? That's prayer at its best—lifting up someone with dignity for her best before the Lord.

Before we ask for prayer for someone, it's good to ask ourselves: Am I perpetuating gossip? Was this prayer request something given to me in confidentiality? Have I tried to imagine what life would be like in this person's shoes? Am I asking out of sincere caring?

If we're not certain if the request was confidential, it's best either to keep the request private or keep the details so hazy it would not embarrass the individual. An example would be, "Lord, protect our teenagers from the influence of alcohol," rather than naming a specific teen's problem. God knows the names and the details.

Recently, while participating in a twenty-four-hour prayer service at my church, I was given a three-by-five card bearing the name of a married couple and the comment "Pray for their marriage." Gulp. That seemed too personal to mention in a setting with six other people, so I prayed for the couple without using their names. I just figured God would know the intent of our hearts anyway. Sometimes that's where all the details should stay—right in our heart.

Prayer Starter

Father, though it's been a hard lesson, thank you for teaching me to keep gossip to myself—even to stop it before it's out of the mouth of someone else. Continue to change my curiosity about others to interest and compassion and to teach me to always pray in love for others. In Jesus' name, amen.

Fitness Tip

If you've been walking for several months or more and have reached a plateau on weight loss, try taking a walk of more than ninety minutes once in a while. Long walks force the body to turn to stored fuel.

Chapter 18

In His Hands

Read 1 Peter 5:1-11.

PRAYERWALK FOCUS
"Humble yourselves therefore under the mighty hand of God, that he may exalt you in due time: Casting all your care upon him; for he careth for you."—1 Peter 5:6-7, KJV

A couple of years ago I was feeling especially burdened by all the concerns I was carrying—illnesses, potential business failure, school personnel problems. Then I sensed God telling me, *So, are you really praying? Are you giving me the concerns? Or do you want to try and handle them yourself?*

Suddenly I realized the arrogance of my prayer posture. I was trying to carry prayer concerns when instead I should have been casting them onto God to carry. Right then I gave the burden to God and again experienced peace as I prayed.

I find it interesting that Peter's admonition to cast our worries on God is tied to the previous verse: "Humble yourselves therefore under the mighty hand of God, that he may exalt you in due time: Casting all your care upon him; for he careth for you" (1 Peter 5:6-7, KJV). It is humbling to acknowledge that we can't fix other people or their problems. I think we sometimes get our Christian ethic mixed up with a Puritan ethic and assume that we have to carry our "fair share of the load." Jesus, however, said his yoke was easy and light and with it we'd find rest for our souls (Matthew 11:28-30). Giving him our cares is the better choice. In giving God our concerns and worries, we are saying that he knows best. We are placing our trust in his power and goodness. "Casting our cares on him" acknowledges that without God we can do nothing.

So how do we *cast* those cares on him? The Greek word for *cast* is *epiripto*, which is used in two senses in the New Testament.[12] It was used in a literal sense in Luke 19:35 when Jesus was entering Jerusalem for the final time. His disciples brought a donkey colt for him to ride, and they *cast* cloaks on the colt and put Jesus on it. The colt would bear the garments, and it would also bear the Lord. But Peter was using *cast* figuratively when he wrote, "casting all your cares." Here *casting* means a placement or discarding of things, an action to get rid of an item. Through prayer we leave our worries and concerns with God.

How can we get to the place where we can give God our concerns? I battled chronic stomachaches from worry until I realized several things. First, God could handle the problem better than I could. Second, my worry over the situation was hurting my witness as a Christian. Others might think my God wasn't big enough to take care of my problems. Third, my hanging on to the problem might have been an impediment to its solution.

I liken this to the story of the little boy who needed to get his bent glasses fixed. He went with his mother to the eye doctor, who agreed they were all out of shape and even hurting his vision. But the little boy didn't want to give them to the doctor, saying, "'Cause I can't see without them." The doctor said, "I can't fix your glasses, son, unless you take them off and give them to me. You'll see better when I'm done." We have to give God our problems and trust that even if we can't see how they'll get fixed, he will do that work better than we can.

We grow in our ability to do this as we practice it, one prayer at a time. It comes down to a matter of trust. We act out of faith. We give our mail to the U.S. Postal Service because we have faith that the workers can do their job and that our mail will get to the right location. And when we give God our concerns, he will deliver the answer just in time—*his* time.

Once we've prayed about our concerns, our burden should be lighter. In a similar vein, Paul wrote,

> Do not be anxious about anything, but in everything, by prayer and petition, with thanksgiving, present your requests to God. And the peace of God, which transcends all understanding, will guard your hearts and your minds in Christ Jesus. (Philippians 4:6-7)

You can cast all your prayers on him because he cares for you.

PRAYER STARTER

Thank you, Father, that you care for us and that with prayer we can cast all our cares upon you. When I try to carry all the burdens of my community, remind me that you do that job much better than I ever could. Thank you for giving me the peace that transcends all my understanding when I pray. In Jesus' name, amen.

FITNESS TIP

For cold weather walking invest in polar fleece clothes. You can wear fewer layers, giving you greater flexibility and freedom of movement.

Chapter 19

On His Wings

DAILY PRAYERWALK
Read Job 42.

PRAYERWALK FOCUS
"My servant Job will pray for you, and I will accept his prayer and not deal with you according to your folly.... After Job had prayed for his friends, the LORD made him prosperous again and gave him twice as much as he had before."—Job 42:8,10

At twenty-one Justin is on a typical post–high school track—get a car, fix up the car, wreck the car, fix up the car… You get the picture. The vehicle is a Chevy Camaro with a T. It has a gorgeous paint job— metallic blue with silver stripes, but it sounds like a Mack truck, approaching and leaving with a roar. My son called this week with the latest news: his third accident. He was okay but had forgotten to make his car insurance payment. So I pray for mercy. His summer job requires that he drive to various locations around the state doing water testing, so he needs his license. But I'm not sure he deserves to keep it, nor am I sure it will be the best thing for him. But I know that God knows, and I'm putting my trust in him as I pray for my son.

I used to mix up the words *grace* and *mercy* until I read Lucinda McDowell's book *Amazed by Grace*. In it she explains that "grace is God's giving us what we don't deserve; mercy is God's not giving us what we do deserve."[13] So I pray for mercy for Justin, who deserves to have his license revoked, and I thank God for gracing him with not just one but two great jobs this summer—with the U.S. Geological Survey and weekends at a golf course (where he'd spend his time anyway).

Many biblical characters also prayed for God's mercy and grace, but Job received both at once. Job was God's proving ground with Satan: God allowed Satan to test Job's faithfulness by sending him a horrible disaster—the loss of his ten children, the devastation of his herds, the death of his servants, and painful sores all over his body. Throughout the test Job did not turn from his God. He complained and questioned God a lot and even wished himself dead, but he never turned his back on God. He remained faithful. He also put up with less-than-helpful litanies from his four friends and responded with human justification and more questions that challenged God's purpose for such things.

Finally God spoke with words that immediately humbled Job:

> Who is this that darkens my counsel
>   with words without knowledge?...
>
> Where were you when I laid the earth's foundation?
>   Tell me, if you understand.
> Who marked off its dimensions? Surely you know! (Job
>   38:2,4-5)

From this we understand a little of what it may take to move God toward mercy. Job was correct in assuming he didn't deserve such a fate;

he was a righteous man. But his questioning of God's motives or plan was not appropriate. In doing so he had offended God and deserved God's judgment. We never find out if Job learned that his losses were part of a heavenly power struggle, one that put Satan in his place. Even so, Job understood that it was enough to know God: He didn't need to know all the whys behind his suffering. He told God, "I know that you can do all things; no plan of yours can be thwarted.… Surely I spoke of things I did not understand, things too wonderful for me to know.… My ears had heard of you but now my eyes have seen you" (42:2,3,5).

When Job saw the Lord, he changed. He said, "Therefore I despise myself and repent in dust and ashes" (verse 6). When we meet God, we, too, will instantly recognize that God is holy and good and that we are not. We have a new perspective of who we are—complaining, unfaithful people who fail in the Trust Department. This awareness evokes repentance and a desire for reconciliation.

God didn't make Job wallow very long. Instead, he chastised three of Job's friends and told Job that if he would pray for them, God, in his mercy, would accept their sacrifice instead of justly punishing them. Job then prayed for his friends—an undeserved kindness after his friends' bullying of him. God accepted Job's prayer and extended both grace and mercy to him. Job received mercy when God did not punish him for his lack of trust. God then graced Job with ten more children, riches and property doubled from before, long life, and the respect and comfort of his family and friends.

Some days I feel as though I'm riding on the wings of God's grace and other days on his mercy. Because of the demands of a job and family and ministry, I'm constantly seeking God's grace to help me keep track of what I need to do and when. And when I lash out at a student, I need God's mercy, so I can make amends and do better the next day.

Our God is a God of grace and mercy. Oh, how we need both! Join me in prayer for mercy and grace in your life and the lives of those you love.

PRAYER STARTER

Oh, Lord, how amazing is your grace and how blessed is your mercy. Thank you for the countless times you have extended both to those I love and to me. I know I can never earn either, Lord, but may I increasingly love you for your graceful touches in my life. In Jesus' name, amen.

FITNESS TIP

When walking, keep your arms bent in a ninety-degree angle. If you want to move at a quicker pace, swing your arms faster, and keep them bent. It may not look graceful, but this technique is the right form.

Chapter 20

We Are Family

DAILY PRAYERWALK
Read John 17.

PRAYERWALK FOCUS
"My prayer is not for them alone. I pray also for those who will believe in me through their message, that all of them may be one, Father, just as you are in me and I am in you. May they also be in us so that the world may believe that you have sent me."—John 17:20-21

The three churches in my little town were making large changes in their ministries when I began prayerwalking. One minister was new. One church had no minister. The third was facing leadership and vision changes. I wanted to pray specifically for these pastors and their congregations, but how?

Then I discovered Jesus' chapter-long prayer in John 17. These twenty-six verses give us a glimpse of how I could pray for these churches, as well as for other ministries.

The prayer is divided into three sections: First, Christ prayed for himself, that he would glorify the Father. Then he prayed for the disciples, for their protection and unity. In the last part of his prayer he prayed for future believers, that they would be unified and would have their heavenly Father's love for one another.

At first it surprised me that Christ's prayer begins with a request for himself. Often when I'm praying for my church, I forget my part in its ministry. When I started prayerwalking past my church each week, I'd pray for each board member and our pastor and other teachers or leaders as though all the responsibility and witness rested with them. I'd forgotten the simple children's chorus I'd learned years ago: "I am the church. You are the church. We are the church *together*." Since I've begun to include myself as part of the church, I've discovered I'm less prone to judge what's happening or not happening there. I'm less critical and more willing to be part of the solution so that my participation brings God glory.

Christ next prayed for his disciples, pleading to his "Holy Father," the only time that address is used in the New Testament. He knew he was about to leave his friends, and so his prayer is a desperate one. Were his followers ready for his sacrifice and the challenges ahead?

He prayed: "Holy Father, protect them by the power of your name...so that they may be one as we are one.... I say these things... so that they may have the full measure of my joy within them.... Protect them from the evil one.... Sanctify them by the truth; your word is truth" (verses 11,13,15,17).

As we pray for our churches, we can pray for protection from being led astray from God, either by our own weaknesses or by the Enemy's diversions. We can also pray for unity, for joy, and for sanctification, that gradual process toward holiness.

But Jesus said his prayer was not only for his disciples, but also for all who would believe. The third part of Jesus' prayer was for future believers. A quickly spreading national ministry that encourages prayer for future believers is Mission America's Lighthouse Movement. Endorsed by hundreds of church denominations and parachurch ministries, its thrust is threefold: prayer, care, share. First we pray for our neighbors, then we demonstrate caring in tangible ways, and then we share our faith. As Jesus prayed for future believers, so can we pray for those around us who do not yet know the Lord.

Jesus knew his life on earth and his ministry were drawing to a close, but his prayers weren't self-focused. Each of his requests was motivated by love. He loved the Father so much that he was yearning to be with him again. He loved his disciples so much that the thought of leaving them broke his heart. He loved those of the world so much that he wanted them all to experience the Father's love.

That both amazes and challenges me. How many times have I prayed for my church out of obligation or desperation or frustration! My prayers often lack the pure love that Christ vulnerably demonstrated in the Upper Room prayer. I get impatient when we spin church program wheels, or I get hurt by some remark. In those times I don't always pray with Christlike vision—the sight that sees beyond the path to the cross to the reunion with the Father. The sight that sees potential rather than human weakness. And the love that sees beyond the motive to the need.

But I'm growing in the right direction. Join me in praying for our churches, ministers, and lay leaders—even yourself. Join me in praying out of love.

PRAYER STARTER

Be glorified in my life, Lord. Be glorified in our church leadership. Protect us, help us live out your Word, and bond us together in your sanctified joy. May we go out into the world as lighthouses, drawing in future believers in love. In Jesus' name, amen.

FITNESS TIP

Avoid overstriding, which can slow you down and increase the risk of injury to your gluteal and hamstring muscles. If you feel a jarring thunk with each heel strike, your stride may be too long.[14] Your stride will lengthen naturally as you pick up speed. Don't force it.

Chapter 21

Two Are Better Than One

DAILY PRAYERWALK
Read Exodus 17:8-16.

PRAYERWALK FOCUS

"Again, I tell you that if two of you on earth agree about anything you ask for, it will be done for you by my Father in heaven. For where two or three come together in my name, there am I with them."—Matthew 18:19-20

When I started prayerwalking, I walked alone. I was fine with that because I figured: Who'd want to get up before five in the morning and walk through snow, rain, or skunk encounters? Besides, I was walking with my Personal Trainer, and I didn't mind being alone with him.

But then one morning I thought I saw a drug deal going down and was subsequently followed. During the same week, a couple of men in a truck hooted at me as they were parked along Main Street. This happened a few weeks later with another truck. I was getting a bit unnerved, and a friend suggested that I'd be safer with a partner.

About that same time I decided to prayerwalk around our town's schools. Some ladies I had met via e-mail were doing just that, and I had sensed God urging me to do the same. However, when I prayerwalked around the elementary school, I grew frustrated that I couldn't always remember the names of the teachers and others who worked there. So I called Pam, who teaches kindergarten and first grade at the school, and asked her to be my prayerwalking partner. We've walked together once a week nearly every week since, and now the staff at the grade school always gets prayed for by name.

God honors joint prayer efforts. "Two are better than one, because they have a good return for their work: If one falls down, his friend can help him up. But pity the man who falls and has no one to help him up!" (Ecclesiastes 4:9-10). Our prayers are more effective when they're echoed with a friend's agreement, and that friend can encourage us to keep on keeping on.

We see this in Exodus 17. The Israelites had been grumbling to Moses about food and water when the Amalekites attacked them. Under Moses' direction, Joshua took some of the men into battle the next day while Moses stood on the hill at Rephidim with his staff and hands raised in petition to God. As long as Moses' hands were raised, the Jews prevailed, but when Moses' hands dropped, the enemy was winning. Moses wouldn't have been able to keep his hands raised in petition. But he had help. When he grew tired, Aaron and Hur sat him down on a rock and held up his hands "one on one side, one on the other—so that his hands remained steady till sunset" (verse 12). That image beautifully pictures what happens when we partner in prayer together. Just as God honored the prayers of Moses, Aaron, and Hur, so he honors our prayers of oneness.

The New Testament also teaches this principle. Jesus taught his disciples that "if two of you on earth agree about anything you ask for, it will be done for you by my Father in heaven. For where two or three come together in my name, there I am with them" (Matthew 18:19-20). This promise has three conditions. First, we have to come together. Second, the two or more pray-ers need to agree about the request. Both of these imply unity. Third, the request should be made in Jesus' name.

Proverbs 27:17 says that as iron sharpens iron, so one friend can sharpen another. Prayerwalking partners can help each other grow in prayer together. As soon as I started prayerwalking with Pam, I noticed how relational her prayers were. She converses with her Father. My prayers were a list of imperative sentences: *Heal Mary. Bless the Joneses' business. Give us your vision.* Listening in on Pam's prayers almost made me feel as though I were hearing one side of an intimate phone conversation.

Pam's prayers are filled with the details of the school's needs and her stories of children and fellow workers. I hang on every word. She also seems to know when something is not right—at school or at church or even in my heart. She'll confront the enemy and take the matter to prayer, and somehow I feel safer when we part ways after an hour or so.

If you haven't found a prayerwalking partner yet, I encourage you to find someone to join you on the streets of your neighborhood. She or he will, literally, double your eyesight.

PRAYER STARTER

Father, I see how even your Son partnered with a dozen disciples. I pray that my prayers will be in agreement with your will as I pray in your Son's name. If you would have me praying with a partner—whether I'm walking or not—please bring us together. In Jesus' name, amen.

Fitness Tip

Walking is practically an injury-free exercise. The most common problem is related to overuse—pushing intensity or distance too soon. Your shins may hurt or your muscles may ache. Remembering the acronym RICE can help you: rest, ice, compression, and elevation. Rest is necessary to let the tissues heal. Ice, compression (with an elastic bandage), and elevation can also reduce inflammation. If the problem persists, see your doctor.

Chapter 22

The Right Focus

Read John 15:1-17.

PRAYERWALK FOCUS
"If you remain in me and my words remain in you, ask whatever you wish, and it will be given you."—John 15:7

Someone recently asked me if I thought prayer alone could keep us close to God. I told her, "No way. It's just as important to study the Bible daily and to worship regularly with other believers."

When I started prayerwalking and began to picture Christ as my Personal Trainer, I developed a hunger to know more about his life— how he reacted, how he spoke, how he prayed. Over several months I read through the gospels several times, then went back through several more times, just reading Christ's quoted words. If he were going to be my Personal Trainer, I wanted to begin to see and think as he would.

So most nights after my kids have gone to bed, I open my Bible, get out a pen, open my journal, read until I feel God has spoken to me, and then write it down. Then I think about it, maybe check other references, read the notes, and write an application for my situation. Studying God's Word corrects and centers my thinking, and I feel I'm growing in his direction.

Jesus taught his disciples about the importance of being connected to him. He was speaking to the disciples, comforting them after informing them that one would betray him and that even Peter would deny him. He goes on to say, "Remain in me, and I will remain in you. No branch can bear fruit by itself; it must remain in the vine. Neither can you bear fruit unless you remain in me.... If you remain in me and my words remain in you, ask whatever you wish, and it will be given you" (John 15:4,7).

Jesus uses the word *remain* (*abide* is used in some versions, from the Greek *meno*) eleven times in this passage. As an English teacher and a writer, I don't use the same word over and over. However, Jesus seems to want us to get the point: *remain!* He wanted the disciples to remain as they were, centered with the Vine and remembering and living by his words. He knew that there were many opportunities for the disciples to fall away if they listened to other influences.

When I study God's Word, I'm "remaining" in Christ and his words. As a result, my desires and thoughts are growing more and more like his. The study of God's Word, partnered with prayerwalking—which has helped me take my eyes off myself and focus them on others—has helped me better represent Christ in my little corner of the world.

This change in me is tested five days a week at my high school, where I teach English, journalism, and creative writing to about 120 teenagers. Staying pleasant and positive all day long is tough. That work is not the hardest for me as a Christian woman though. The more difficult challenge is staying pleasant and positive after three o'clock each workday—when the final school bell rings and I go home to be a mom and wife after an exhausting day.

A few days ago I got a glimpse of God's graceful working in me when Bethany burst into the computer room at 2:55 P.M. My creative writing students were still bringing me their poems to critique because we were on a production deadline. Every moment counted, but there was Bethany: "Mom, can I go over to Alexis's house because she…"

Ordinarily I would have answered sharply something like, "Go to my classroom, and wait for me there!"

But this time I saw a little girl who simply had a need. So I gave her a hug, said hello, and asked her to let me finish my class first. Later we went over to her friend's house together. Change from the inside out.

To know God's will and become more like Christ, we need to study God's Word faithfully. Here are a few suggestions for getting started.

- Read straight through the Bible. *Discipleship Journal* prints a schedule you can follow to finish in a year in its December issue. You can download the reading schedule through the magazine's Web site (www.navpress.com/dj_brp.asp) or order it or the magazine by calling 1-800-366-7788.

- Read the Bible in chronological order. The American Tract Society prints a guide called *Through the Bible in a Year!* that offers one reading guide.[15] I taught a Sunday school class that used this guide to study the whole Bible in a year, and it was a year of tremendous growth for me.

- Use a devotional Bible for a daily reading plan and accompanying devotion.

- Bible study books can help keep you focused. You can set a goal of studying all the gospels, for example, and get Bible studies at a Christian bookstore that will help guide you.

- Read different versions of the Bible. Right now I'm reading through the New Testament in Eugene Peterson's *The Message,* which brings us Scripture in language we use today.

We are blessed with so many ways we can take in God's Word. Certainly I can find a way and a time that work for me...and so can you.

PRAYER STARTER

Dear Father, forgive me when I choose not to remain in you by neglecting the study of your Word. Help me set aside significant time each day to systematically read the Bible. Help me abide in Christ and your Word so that my prayers are effective and so that my life is as well. In Jesus' name, amen.

FITNESS TIP

It's hard to stick with walking when your shin muscles hurt. In *Walking: A Complete Guide to the Complete Exercise,* Casey Meyers recommends that when you're experiencing shin muscle aches to continue to "walk at a speed that causes discomfort in the muscle, hold it as long as you can, then slow down to a pace where the discomfort disappears. Walk at that pace for about half the distance you just walked when the shin was uncomfortable, then pick up the pace and fatigue the muscle again."[16] Meyers says this is called progression and overload and that over time the muscle will get stronger.

Chapter 23

Friendship Factor

DAILY PRAYERWALK
Read Revelation 3:14-22.

PRAYERWALK FOCUS
"Here I am! I stand at the door and knock. If anyone hears my voice and opens the door, I will come in and eat with him, and he with me."—Revelation 3:20

My friend June and I do everything together. Study the Bible. Sit next to each other in church. Scout the local antique stores. Fix each other tea when life clouds over. A couple of years ago I even talked her into prayerwalking with me twice a week. She has so many interests and is so interesting herself that others rarely guess she's old enough to be my mom.

My day rarely seems complete until I've talked with June on the phone. I usually call her while I'm fixing dinner or cleaning up dishes and unload all my day's joys and junk on her. Although she's busy with her own writing projects, volunteer work, and family, she's never too busy for me. It's not infrequent for me to call her with an urgent prayer need or a request to run an errand. She always says, "Sure! I can do that!" She always has time for me, and I think it's our daily conversation that has cemented our friendship.

June's giving friendship gives me a concrete picture of how God can be a friend to me. He is ready at a thought's notice to hear from us and to speak to us as well. His passionate interest in us is seen in Revelation 3:20: "Here I am! I stand at the door and knock. If anyone hears my voice and opens the door, I will come in and eat with him, and he with me." He is always available, always waiting for us to call out for help, direction, or companionship.

Some might say this is a bit presumptuous—to call God "friend"—but Scripture sets a precedent for this. In Isaiah 41:8 God called Abraham "my friend." This is echoed in King Jehoshaphat's prayer when he recalled that God had given the land to "Abraham your friend" (2 Chronicles 20:7).

Let's look at this friendship. In Genesis 18 when the Lord, accompanied by two angels, visited Abraham at his tent, the Lord said, "I will surely return to you about this time next year, and Sarah your wife will have a son" (verse 10). Abraham ministered to the visitors' physical needs and then "walked along with them to see them on their way" (verse 16). The Lord said, "Shall I hide from Abraham what I am about to do?" (verse 17) and then told him that he would be the father of a powerful nation. When the Lord told his friend that Sodom and Gomorrah would be destroyed for their sin, Abraham negotiated with God in an attempt to spare the two cities from judgment.

We see several characteristics of a great friendship in this story. One friend humbles himself and serves his visitors. The other friend grants a long-term request, and then the two dialogue—speaking, listening, seeing each other's point of view, and agreeing.

We can have a similar kind of relationship with God as well. It just requires our initiative. God wants a meaningful relationship with us, but he's not going to push down the door. Certainly, it's clear that he welcomes our prayer visits, since he is the one who is knocking at our door, the one who had the idea of a personal relationship in the first place. But as a friend said recently, "He's a gentleman. He won't push himself or his ways on us." He wants us to open the door. When I'm walking and talking with God, seeking him out daily, choosing him over other activities, it's my hope that he sees me as his friend, just as he did Abraham.

Some days I don't feel like a very good friend at all. When I open the front door to prayerwalk, sometimes I start with, "I don't feel like praying, Lord." But even on those days I find that, like June, he is available, listens to my junk, and reminds me of his love for me through a remembrance of his faithful work in my life or a scripture verse.

Yesterday I was walking as the early November sky broke into dawn's colors. As the pinks and purples crept across the eastern sky, God silently whispered, *My love for you endures forever.* Jesus loves me; this I know.

PRAYER STARTER

Father, help me to never take my relationship with you for granted. I want to know you more and to be worthy to be called your friend. I want nothing else to take your place, and I thank you that when I approach you each new day, you delight in my seeking of you. In Jesus' name, amen.

FITNESS TIP

Prevention's Practical Encyclopedia of Walking for Health offers the following suggestions if you're threatened by a dog:[17]

- Put a stick or something between the dog and yourself.
- Assert authority with a "Go home!" or some other command.
- Avoid eye contact.
- Use a commercial dog repellent spray.

For a pesky dog I encounter on one route, I have a two-by-four hidden, which I pick up and carry when I cross his path. Another tactic I've used with dogs is to pick up a small stick and throw it, pretending I'm playing a game.

Chapter 24

Listening for His Voice

DAILY PRAYERWALK
Read 1 Samuel 3:1–4:1.

PRAYERWALK FOCUS

"The LORD came and stood there, calling as at the other times, 'Samuel! Samuel!' Then Samuel said, 'Speak, for your servant is listening.'"—1 Samuel 3:10

Samuel, whose mother had dedicated him to godly service as a boy, worked in the temple at Shiloh under the priestly judge Eli. One night the Lord called out Samuel's name three times, but he didn't recognize the voice of God because he "did not yet know the LORD" (1 Samuel 3:7). Eli figured out what was happening and told Samuel that the next time God called, to say, "Speak, LORD, for your servant is listening" (verse 9). The fourth time was the charm, and God gave Samuel an important message—a condemnation of the house of Eli. It must have taken great courage for Samuel to tell this to the mentor who had raised him, yet he did. He had heard God speak.

Although Samuel started out as a boy who couldn't recognize God's voice, he learned to hear it and lived out his godly purpose as a priest and judge. Samuel became the last of the heroes of the premonarchical age and the first of the prophets who stood alongside the kings. Like Eli, he was also a judge, leading the Jews in his area. He stepped aside when the people began calling for a king to lead them, anointing Saul and then rejecting him when Saul's heart turned against God. Samuel then anointed David, the ancestor and foreshadower of Jesus Christ. When Samuel died, all Israel assembled and mourned (1 Samuel 25:1).

In the Bible God communicated to his people in many different ways. An angel brought God's good news to Mary (Luke 1:26-38). Daniel saw visions. Jacob heard from God through dreams (Genesis 28:10-19). The glory of God was revealed to Ezekiel (Ezekiel 8). Jeremiah understood he was clay in God's hands when he saw a potter working (Jeremiah 18:1-10). God spoke to Elijah through a gentle whisper (1 Kings 19:12-13). The many miracles of Christ spoke of God's power.

God still speaks to us today. In *Experiencing God,* Henry Blackaby and Claude King say that God can speak to us through the Bible, through other believers, through circumstances, and through prayer.[18] God wants us to still our hearts, open our eyes, attune our ears—to wait, look, and listen. In prayer we converse with God, and just as we listen when we converse with a friend, so we need to listen to God in prayer.

Every week I try to devote most of one prayerwalking session to listening for God's word to me. I invite God to speak, and then I wait for his voice. Blackaby writes that "when God speaks, it is to reveal something about Himself, His purposes, or His ways. God's revelations are designed to bring you into a love relationship with Him."[19] I've found this to be true in my own life. When God speaks to me—usually with inaudible, simple, direct words—he often directs me to a new understanding of him or life or a new course of action. As I rely on him for direction and guidance, this practice is now as essential to me as breathing.

My ability to recognize God's voice has increased with my growing understanding and knowledge of Scripture. As I've read about God's persistent pursuit of a love relationship with humanity—with me— my desire to get to know him and to listen to his voice has deepened.

And he *has* spoken to me. When I first asked God whether to take a sabbatical, he answered, "Not yet." Later he spoke to me through the encouragement of other believers: "Go for it!" When I told him of the pain I felt over a broken relationship, he reminded me that he loves me and that this breach didn't happen for my discipline but because he's pruning me in preparation for a greater task that lies ahead. ("Consider it all joy, Janet, when you encounter various trials…") He guides me with a quiet sense or nudge of sorts when I'm prayerwalking, and often I encounter a situation or person who needs prayer ("Walk by the church.")

God's first words to Samuel were, "See, I am about to do something in Israel that will make the ears of everyone who hears of it tingle" (1 Samuel 3:11). I have found that every time God speaks to me, not only my ears but also my whole body tingles. Just imagine: You could hear from the Lord Most High today. What a privilege!

PRAYER STARTER

Dear Lord, it is hard to imagine that you'd want to talk to me. May I live my life today with my ear turned toward you. Help me remember that it's more important for me to hear from you than it is for you to hear from me. Direct my thoughts and quiet my heart enough so that I may clearly hear your voice. In Jesus' name, amen. [20]

FITNESS TIP

If you walk during the daytime, wear a sunscreen that blocks both UVA and UVB rays. The words "broad spectrum" should be on the label. If you're after a tan, try a lotion with skin tint. I use Coppertone Oil Free Effortless Color Sunless Tanning Lotion. It really does work, and I've gotten compliments on my "great tan."

Chapter 25

Watch and Pray

DAILY PRAYERWALK
Read Mark 14:32-42.

PRAYERWALK FOCUS

"Could you not keep watch for one hour? Watch and pray so that you will not fall into temptation. The spirit is willing, but the body is weak."—Mark 14:37-38

For most of my adult life I have struggled with my weight. The exercise I get from prayerwalking helps, but I still have a weakness for some favorite foods—cookies, breads, anything chocolate. When my life is especially busy, I'm tempted to turn to food for comfort. I've even deluded myself into believing that carbohydrates, such as microwave popcorn, M&M's, or Jelly Bellies, help force out the creative juices. Hmm…I should instead remember that prayer has worked better as I'm searching for the right words. And prayer is a key as we turn away from temptation.

Jesus recommended prayer as a guard against temptation in the Gethsemane garden. After the Upper Room meal he told his twelve disciples not only that one of them would betray him, but that they *all* would fall away. When Peter declared that he wouldn't do such a thing, Jesus said Peter would disown him three times before the rooster crowed that night. Judas had already left to inform the chief priests where to find the man who said he was God.

So when Jesus and his disciples entered into the garden area on the Mount of Olives, he asked Peter, James, and John to be with him and keep watch as he prayed. He moved away from them and prayed awhile, and when he returned, he found them sleeping. "Could you not keep watch for one hour?" he asked. "Watch and pray so that you will not fall into temptation. The spirit is willing, but the body is weak."

Isn't this the truth? Our spirits are willing, but our bodies are weak.

I don't fault the disciples for falling asleep. They'd had a rough day. They'd had the emotional dinner in the Upper Room when Jesus had said, "This is my body.... This is my blood." The disciples even argued about which one of them was the greatest (Luke 22:24). Perhaps it was then that Christ chose to wash their feet (John 13:3-17). Any one of those segments of their evening meal would have been emotionally challenging, so much so that after their strenuous hike up the Mount of Olives, they must have been exhausted.

I know what it's like to doze off while praying; that's one reason I started prayerwalking. However, prayer is a crucial component as we face those things that tempt us. I know what it's like to start a new diet, only to see it fall away, because I've tried to muster my own strength to work my way through it. I often fail, looking to food for a temporary fix instead of going to God.

Prayer is our greatest weapon for fighting temptation. When we're praying, we're focused on seeking what God wants, what God can do, and who God is. Because God is omnipotent, he can give us the power to resist temptation. When Jesus was at what may have been his weakest moment—"Take this cup from me"—he went to his Father in prayer. In prayer, then, he decided, "Yet not what I will, but what you will" (Mark 14:36).

What you will. That simple prayer may be all we need at those times when we're tempted to act out of sinfulness rather than Christlikeness. We can pray *what you will* when we're tempted to pass on some gossip. We can pray *what you will* in the line at the grocery store when someone cuts in line in front of us and we want to lash out in irritation and anger. We can pray *what you will* when we're tempted to sleep in instead of spending time alone with God in prayer.

Jesus has given us an important two-step directive when facing those things in life that can trip us up as Christians. Watch out in awareness, then pray. After all, we're in training.

Prayer Starter

Father, you are worthy of my all-day-long attention. Help me readjust my thinking and my priorities so that I can spend wakeful, purposeful time with you each day. Teach me to watch and pray so that I don't give in to temptation. In Jesus' name, amen.

Fitness Tip

In *Fitness Walking for Women* Anne Kashiwa and James Rippe, M.D., offer a twenty-week low-level fitness program that can help you build from a thirty-minute, one-mile workout (including five-minute warmup and cool-down periods) to a one-hour, three-mile workout (including the same warmup and cool-down time).[21] Basically, you slowly add a little distance and time, then add intensity in the same number of minutes, then repeat the process until you're walking three miles in forty-five minutes, plus the warmup and cool-down times.

Chapter 26

Give Me Wisdom, Father

DAILY PRAYERWALK
Read 1 Kings 3:1-15.

PRAYERWALK FOCUS
"So give your servant a discerning heart to govern your people and to distinguish between right and wrong. For who is able to govern this great people of yours?"—1 Kings 3:9

It was eight days until the day our Rebekah married her Ozzie. Somehow she and I had survived ten months of shopping, planning, deciding, arguing, crying, apologizing. We'd made it until the final countdown, contracts and feelings intact. She'd made it through student teaching and her senior year of college. I'd made it through a year of teaching, writing, interviewing, and raising kids. All the wedding details were falling into place, and all was well—until the phone call. I'd been making final lists: To Do, To Buy, To Take.

"Honey, do you want me to get the unity candle?" I asked.

No, they wanted to pick it out.

"How about the candle base?"

Sure.

"Oh, I got a garter—is that okay?"

Oh…was it blue?

"Umm…no—but it's prettier. The blue one looked cheesy."

Okay. Fine.

A few yeses and noes later we hung up. Rebekah had said that everything was fine. But somehow it wasn't.

I was flying down almost a week ahead of time, both to help my daughter and to attend a three-day speakers' conference in the Los Angeles area so that I could learn more about speaking professionally. I had thought—in my normal, efficient manner—that I could accomplish two things at once. But after our phone call I sensed that Rebekah felt hurt and frustrated that I wasn't coming just to be with her at this significant time in her life. Maybe we needed some time together…but how could that be arranged with my conference already scheduled and paid for?

Give me wisdom, Father, I prayed as the sun crept over the mountaintop. And he did, through my friend Susan. When I got home and logged on to my e-mail, I read her message:

> If you feel stressed, you might want to ask if you can postpone your class. They have them yearly…. I just can't imagine how you could (attend the seminar)…. A wedding is right up there with the stresses of death and divorce.

Wow! Susan's wise words made the light go on. I called the seminar's office and became the first registrant for the following year. Instantly peace reigned throughout my entire being. When I called Rebekah, she was delighted that she'd have my complete attention the week before her wedding.

How much pain, suffering, and embarrassment could we save ourselves if we made it a daily—in fact, a constant—practice to pray for God's wisdom before acting? James wrote, "If any of you lacks wisdom, he should ask God, who gives generously to all without finding fault, and it will be given to him" (James 1:5).

Not only does God grant us wisdom when we ask for it, but he gives it generously. When God told King Solomon that he could have whatever he wanted, Solomon asked for a discerning heart to govern God's people and "to distinguish between right and wrong" (1 Kings 3:9). The Bible records that God was so pleased with the request that he granted Solomon not only wisdom but also riches and honor (1 Kings 3:13). Later when Solomon resolved the maternity issue of the baby claimed by two women, all Israel "held the king in awe, because they saw that he had wisdom from God to administer justice (verse 28).

God was generous with me as well. When I told another friend about Bekah's reaction to the garter I had bought, she secretly made a blue one that was much more beautiful than the one I had purchased for $6.95 plus tax…and she jokingly charged me fifty cents, which I gladly and laughingly paid.

Also, every single minute of my time with my daughter was taken up with errand running, which was all worth it when she put her arms around me and said, "Thanks, Mom. It was just great." But I didn't need her words. The dream-come-true look in my daughter's eyes said it all.

I have a postscript on the conference too. As it turned out, my flight was canceled, and I would have missed most of the first morning's presentation!

Prayer Starter

Dear Father, thank you for overlooking my unwise past decisions and meting out wisdom when I seek you. Thank you also that your wisdom is right at my fingertips within the pages of your Word as well as through the counsel of your people. Help me to seek you first with every breath and step I take. In Jesus' name, amen.

FITNESS TIP

You've heard that it's a good idea to let your car warm up before you drive off. The same is true for your body. You'll tax your heart unnecessarily if you just start off at an aerobic pace. Move at a slower pace for about five minutes, then work into your aerobic zone.

Chapter 27

Greater Than Any of Our Fears

DAILY PRAYERWALK
Read 2 Chronicles 20:1-30.

PRAYERWALK FOCUS
"Jehoshaphat was afraid and turned his attention to seek the LORD, and proclaimed a fast throughout all Judah."—2 Chronicles 20:3, NASB

Jehoshaphat had good, human reason to be afraid. Three nations had joined to fight against this king of Judah, the southern kingdom, and his men had told him a vast army was approaching. If you or I were he, what would we do? Meet with our generals? Round up the charioteers? Enlist all able men? Run?

All of these are likely choices, but Jehoshaphat did none of them.

When the news brought fear to his heart, he "resolved to inquire of the LORD" (verse 3). The men who had warned Jehoshaphat of the coming armies must have been panicked. Perhaps they were even offering advice. But instead of continuing to listen to their worries, he changed spiritual posture and did two immediate actions—he determined to seek the Lord and proclaimed a fast throughout all Judah.

The people came from every town in Judah and banded together with their godly king, praying that God would help them.

The people came to the temple in Jerusalem, where Jehoshaphat prayed for God's help. The prayer was succinct and faith-filled. He reminded God of what he had done in the past. Instead of moaning and groaning about what awful possibility was ahead, Jehoshaphat simply recited what he knew: that God was all-powerful, that God would hear and save them, and that the people would look to God alone.

In response, God went to battle for these people who had chosen to praise and honor him with their prayers. He created confusion in the three opposing armies, and they ended up slaughtering each other. The men of Judah immediately headed to the temple to praise God with their harps and lutes and trumpets. But the story didn't end there: All the neighboring kingdoms got wind of God's victory in Judah, and peace reigned for the rest of Jehoshaphat's twenty-five-year reign.

We, too, can dismantle our fear when we turn our attention away from the situation and immediately seek God's guidance and help through prayer. It's easy to get hung up on what we think is the only reality—the threat. The greater reality is that God is all-powerful, he will hear our prayers, and we can trust him for what seems impossible. Trusting God with our fears, however, doesn't mean we won't have to face them. When Elijah was running for his life after Queen Jezebel's threats to have him killed, God told him, "Go back the way you came" (1 Kings 19:15). Elijah ran because he felt powerless against the wicked queen's influence. However, with God's help he was protected. We have to face our fears, but if we turn to God first, we have his help when we eventually face them down.

When I began prayerwalking, I was afraid of the dark. But every day my Personal Trainer and I faced the darkness and walked through it. Eventually my heart only pounded from the workout, not the anxiety. When I realized I'd overcome my fear of the dark, I decided to challenge other fears I'd had. As a child I'd had nightmares of falling and was afraid of heights in the daytime, too. A year ago when I visited Colorado Springs, I drove to the top of Pike's Peak in a tiny rental car. The road ascends eight thousand feet, winding around very tight corners on the edge of precipitous cliffs. In fact, many of those drop-offs may have been thousands of feet. But I made it to the top, admittedly a little shaky. At the gift store at the 14,110-foot peak, I selected the T-shirt that would announce to the world that I had made it up and took it to a young man at a register.

"Do you ever have people who drive up here and can't go back down?" I asked.

He leaned over and whispered, "Are you one of those people?"

"Maybe," I whispered back.

When he told me I could make it back—in low gear—I decided maybe I *wasn't* one of those people. And I wasn't. Afterward I even climbed the 224 steps of the suspended staircase of Seven Falls—and back down in a lightning storm! Okay, I did hold up quite a few folks behind me going down, but...*I made it!*

Our God is greater than our fears.

PRAYER STARTER

Dear Father, thank you that you are all-powerful. You are stronger than any force that would threaten me or keep me from boldly pursuing your will in my life. Thank you that you hear me when I call. I love knowing that you delight in my seeking you. Help me, Lord, to turn from that which would make me fall and to turn toward you. In Jesus' name, amen.

FITNESS TIP

You may want to add resistance training to your routine to help stave off bone-mass loss and osteoporosis. These include the following exercises: squats, walking lunges, or standing weighted leg lifts for your lower body, and push-ups, tricep dips, or pull-ups for your upper body.[22]

Chapter 28

When God Says No

Read 2 Corinthians. 12:1-10.

PRAYERWALK FOCUS
"Three times I pleaded with the Lord to take it away from me. But he said to me, 'My grace is sufficient for you, for my power is made perfect in weakness.'"—2 Corinthians 12:8-9

A month after I began prayerwalking, we learned that my dad was diagnosed with amyotrophic lateral sclerosis, commonly called Lou Gehrig's Disease. He was already beginning to lose control of his muscles: He could hardly swing a golf club, and Mom had started mowing their lawn. Naturally, when my mom and we five kids learned about Dad's ALS, we began praying for healing. Just a little over five months later, though, he was gone, and part of our grieving process involved the age-old questions, *Why didn't God heal my dad? Why did he answer no?*

After all, didn't Jesus tell his disciples that they could ask for anything, and that they would receive their answer in joy (John 16:24)? Yes…but the day after he said these words, Jesus went to the Garden of

Gethsemane and prayed, "Take this cup from me" (Mark 14:36). An hour later, he was arrested and headed for the cross. On the cross he prayed, "My God, my God, why have you forsaken me?" (Mark 15:34). God answered no to Jesus' prayers—and we know that Jesus was full of faith and had the mind of God when he prayed! Obviously, Jesus must have been giving the disciples a principle, not an absolute promise when he told them, "Ask and you will receive, and your joy will be complete" (John 16:24).

But wait a minute. Did you catch the last phrase of that verse? *And your joy will be complete.* Could it be that Jesus was saying that God's answer would bring *joy,* not that God would do what we ask?

That certainly seemed to be true for Paul. Three times he pleaded with God to take away what he called "a thorn in my flesh" (2 Corinthians 12:7-8). Theologians have speculated about what his infirmity could have been—malaria, epilepsy, eye trouble, migraine headaches, or something else. Despite the apostle's prayers, God said no.

Most of us have a hard time with *no.* We think we know what's best, or we may view a negative answer as a rejection of ourselves. But not Paul. A strong personality, he wrote that his physical problem was keeping him from becoming conceited. Christ had told him, "My grace is sufficient for you, for my power is made perfect in weakness" (verse 9).

Paul found it possible to find joy even when God said no. He wrote that his infirmity gave him even that much more opportunity to do his work in weakness so that he would have to rely on Christ's power. Paul said that this opportunity to testify to Christ's strength gave him the chance to delight "in weaknesses, in insults, in hardships, in persecutions, in difficulties" (verse 10). Our strength as Christians paradoxically comes from our weakness. When we have to rely on the power of God, we display the work of divine power in our lives.

Knowing this may not make it any easier as we're facing the death of a child, a divorce, a job layoff, or some other loss. Knowing that others, including Christ, have suffered may not erase the whys of our lives. But when God says no, he longs to comfort us through other Christians. When Paul was suffering with his illness, the Galatians welcomed him and cared for him. Later he wrote them, saying, "If you could have done so, you would have torn out your eyes and given them to me" (Galatians 4:15).

Good things can come from a no answer…things that can lead to joy. We can learn to rely on God's grace. We can learn to identify with Christ in suffering. Our hardships give others the opportunity to serve. Struggles can keep our egos in check. Ultimately, God can be glorified through our weakness.

My dad demonstrated this truth. Lou Gehrig's disease can take away a man's dignity: You eventually have to have someone feed you and take care of all your physical needs. Dad did that with grace and humor. He showed the world around him how a Christian man can face death with faith and dignity. Like Paul, Dad was at his strongest when he was at his weakest. When we are faced with struggles, we, too, can show others that our faith makes a difference, for God's grace will still be sufficient.

PRAYER STARTER

Father, I know that I don't always know what's best for me, but sometimes it's hard when you tell me no. Teach me how to accept that response from you gracefully and also to delight in it. Help me live out my faith in such a way that your power is made perfect through my weaknesses. In Jesus' name, amen.

FITNESS TIP

To breathe correctly while walking aerobically, breathe deeply, expanding your stomach. In this way your lungs will fill completely, and your body will get more oxygen.

Chapter 29

Overboard and Desperate

DAILY PRAYERWALK
Read Jonah 2.

PRAYERWALK FOCUS
"Then Jonah prayed to the LORD his God from the stomach of the fish, and he said, 'I called out of my distress to the LORD, and He answered me. I cried for help from the depth of Sheol; You heard my voice.'"—Jonah 2:1-2, NASB

After my father's death I hid a lot. Sleep was my refuge. I had spent my adrenaline, I guess, on the hurried two-hour trip to the hospital when I heard he would probably not make it through the night. When I got there and found Dad gone, I had a hard time facing God, but in sleep I could forget Dad was gone and could enter some other temporary reality.

Humanity has a history of hiding from God. The prophet Jonah tried to run away from God when he didn't like what God was telling him. When God called Jonah to travel five hundred miles from home to preach to the city of Nineveh, he got on a boat and headed in the other direction. God, however, can find us in our hiding places, and when God brought a great storm, Jonah told the crew that the storm was his fault and that they should throw him over. A great fish swallowed him whole, and Jonah managed to survive in the fish's belly for three days and three nights.

Finally… "*Then* Jonah prayed…from the stomach of the fish" (Jonah 2:1, NASB, emphasis added). Apparently, he continued to avoid God for three days before he cried out to him, as we have no record that he prayed when God called him to Nineveh, when he ran, when he boarded the ship for Tarshish, when the Lord sent a great storm, or when he admitted his sin before the crew and was thrown overboard. All we know is that Jonah prayed when he felt he was on the edge of death: "From the depths of the grave I called for help, and you listened to my cry" (verse 2). He waited until the last possible moment before calling for God's help. Perhaps he was ashamed or felt that he had gotten himself into the situation and had to get himself out.

In any case, Jonah finally prayed. His prayer is a piecemeal collection of verses from Psalms.[23] It's a beautiful eight-verse prayer thanking God for disciplining him, expressing his faith in God's rescue, and promising to sacrifice to the Lord. This prayer models for us the value of memorizing Scripture so that when we're without words of our own, we can fall back on God's Word to form what we need to pray.

It's also a strong model of how Scripture memory can help build our faith. Jonah was certain that God would save him from otherwise certain death. We see this when he prayed, "Salvation comes from the LORD" (verse 9). His patchwork prayer of psalms reflects expectancy. Jonah knew that God was listening. He knew salvation only comes from God. He also knew that God would redeem him. He recognized the whole bizarre incident as part of God's plan for his life, a discipline. Even though the sailors literally tossed Jonah into the water, he recognized that action also was God's plan. (*"You* hurled me into the deep"—verse 3, emphasis added.) As soon as Jonah finished his prayer, God directed the fish to vomit Jonah up onto the beach; from there he headed for Nineveh and fulfilled his original call to preach.

When we are desperate, God hears us and will help us in our struggle…even if our desperation has arisen out of disobedience or avoidance of God.

After a few days of hiding from God, I realized that I was avoiding the only One who could truly comfort me in my loss. I confessed my anger with God for not healing my father. I made a conscious decision to embrace his will and put on my sweats and walking shoes and headed out the door, praying, "O Lord, my Lord, how excellent is your name in all the earth! When I consider the moon and the stars, the work of your hands, what is man that you are mindful of him?" (adapted from Psalm 8:1-4).

Fill your memory with psalms, and when you're in the depth of despair and cannot form a prayer of your own, God's words will fill your heart, giving you the comfort or wisdom you so desperately need.

PRAYER STARTER

Redeemer God, thank you that you hear my cries, even when I've run in the opposite direction of you. Thank you for pursuing me even when I'm not choosing to obey your call or follow you. Help me fill my memory with psalms so that even when I cannot phrase my own prayer, your Word will just naturally flow out of my being. Thank you, God, that you give me second and third and many more chances. I pray that I am worthy of your call. In Jesus' name, amen.

FITNESS TIP

Vary your prayerwalking route. We live in an evil world, and if our routine becomes too predictable, we can fall into someone's awful and hurtful plan. Let your family know, however, where you intend to walk and how long you will be gone. Carrying a cell phone is a good idea too, and identification is a must. Just be careful and aware.

Chapter 30

Changing God's Mind

DAILY PRAYERWALK
Read Jonah 3.

PRAYERWALK FOCUS
"When God saw what they did and how they turned from their evil ways, he had compassion and did not bring upon them the destruction he had threatened."—Jonah 3:10

All of my children are experts in the art of persuasion, especially Bethany, age ten. She recently forgot to ask her father's permission before making a commitment with a friend, so Craig told her she couldn't go over to friends' houses for a month. But when Chelsea, Bethany's friend since birth, moved, they wanted to spend time together with the third cord of the friendship strand, Emily. After Bethany made her strong case with her dad, he relented. Why? It was a special case, but most of all, Bethany's heart had changed. She didn't argue with Craig; she was ready to accept his answer, no matter what it was.

Just as Bethany's change of heart influenced Craig to change his mind, our hearts can influence God to change his mind as well.

When King David and his army began to rely on numbers of fighting men instead of on God, God sent a plague that killed seventy thousand people. When David understood what was happening, he asked God to punish him and his family instead of the people and immediately began to build an altar to the Lord. *"Then* the LORD answered prayer in behalf of the land, and the plague on Israel was stopped" (2 Samuel 24:25, emphasis added). David had stopped relying on the might of his army and had put his trust in God again—and God withdrew his intended punishment.

David's heart had changed, so God changed his mind.

God also changed his mind about destroying the people of Nineveh. He called Jonah to tell the city of Nineveh that God was going to destroy the city in forty days. To Jonah's dismay, "the Ninevites believed God" (Jonah 3:5). When the king of Nineveh heard Jonah's prophecy, he sent out a decree, stating:

> Let man and beast be covered with sackcloth. Let everyone
> call urgently on God. Let them give up their evil ways and their
> violence. Who knows? God may yet relent and with compassion
> turn from his fierce anger so that we will not perish.
> (verses 8-9)

When God saw their change of heart, "he had compassion and did not bring upon them the destruction he had threatened" (verse 10).

God can change his mind—when we demonstrate a changed heart.

When God told Abraham that he was going to destroy the cities of Sodom and Gomorrah, Abraham pleaded with God to save Sodom if there were fifty righteous men in the city. Then Abraham persuaded God to agree to save the city if there were forty-five, then forty, then thirty, then twenty, and finally ten righteous men. (Abraham may have figured there were at least ten in his family.) But when Abraham couldn't point to ten people who were righteous, God did what he said he would do and destroyed both cities.

In this instance, God didn't change his mind, but according to Jesus, he would have if the people had repented. When Jesus was condemning the people of Capernaum for their unbelief, he told them: "If the miracles that were performed in you had been performed in Sodom, it would have remained to this day" (Matthew 11:23). In other words, God would have changed his mind if the people had changed.

At times we can be tempted to think what will be will be, that God is going to do what he's going to do, so what is the point of praying? Nothing could be further from the truth. The previous examples show us that we can influence—change—God's intentions by our actions and our prayers. While these passages show God as changing his mind about judging people for their sins, James tells us that this principle is broader than that. Some things won't happen unless we ask God for them—"You do not have, because you do not ask God" (James 4:2). And in Exodus 32:11,14 we read: "But Moses sought the favor of the LORD his God. 'O LORD,' he said, 'why should your anger burn against your people, whom you brought out of Egypt with great power and a mighty hand?'… Then the LORD relented and did not bring on his people the disaster he had threatened." In this instance God changed his mind because of Moses' sincere prayer—even though the people's hearts had not changed.

Our prayers matter—that is why we pray.

PRAYER STARTER

Thank you, God, first for hearing our prayers. Thank you also that you would consider our pleas—in all their humanness—and answer them, even change your plans sometimes, Lord. Teach me to be as merciful toward others as you are—extending touches of grace throughout my day. In Jesus' name, amen.

Fitness Tip

DON'T wear all-cotton socks when prayerwalking. Synthetics help socks stay soft and resilient and even help prevent blisters. It's better to wear socks with a little nylon or Spandex.

Before We Even Ask...

Read Daniel 9:20-27.

PRAYERWALK FOCUS
"Before they call I will answer; while they are still speaking I will hear."—Isaiah 65:24

Around nine o'clock one winter morning a few years ago, my friend Sharon called me in a panic while I was at a prayer-partner meeting at church. Her oldest child, Crystal, had called at one o'clock, Texas time, the previous morning to let her mom know that her car had broken down while she was driving back to college. Crystal hadn't known what to do, and so she walked three miles down the highway to a little town called Van Buren, leaving her dogs and pet ducks in her pickup truck. Sharon hadn't heard from her daughter since the night before and didn't even know where to begin looking for her.

When I heard this, I interrupted the meeting, and twenty or more of us prayed for Crystal—for protection, for help with her truck, for a safe place to stay, and for a quick phone call to her mom!

Sharon called me again about an hour later. Just as she had hung up with me, Crystal's dorm mother, Hazel, called to find out where Crystal was. Sharon told her about Crystal's phone call. As it turned out, Hazel was from the little town of Van Buren, Texas, and knew everyone there—the tow-truck driver, the sheriff, the motel owner. Soon Sharon talked to the sheriff and learned that Crystal had had her truck towed and repaired in the night, had gotten a motel room with the tow-truck driver's help, and was on her way to her college in Abilene at that very moment.

When I told Sharon the specific prayers we had prayed, she said, "God knew you would be praying and had already answered the very prayers you prayed."

I had never heard this before—that God could answer our prayers before we even thought of them. But Scripture supports this belief. The Lord told Isaiah, "Before they call I will answer; while they are still speaking I will hear" (Isaiah 65:24). Earlier in Isaiah it says that the Lord "longs to be gracious to you," that he rises to show us compassion and will answer as soon as he hears (Isaiah 30:18-19). In his Sermon on the Mount, Jesus said that the Father knows what we need before we ask him (Matthew 6:8).

We know what this is like. When we're in conversation with people we know well, we'll complete their sentences, beating that person to the punch. As parents and friends we often sense what our child or friend needs and take care of the request before it's even made. How much more is our Father a caring parent, who often takes care of those needs before we're even aware of them?

Daniel also experienced God's answers to his prayers before they were fully uttered. The prophet was serving the Babylonian king Darius, one of at least four he would serve there. He had gained the king's respect after God had protected him in the lion's den, and the king had issued a decree that everyone in the nation must fear and reverence Daniel's God (Daniel 6:26). Daniel was fasting and praying and petitioning and pleading that God would be merciful about judgment against Jerusalem when the angel Gabriel interrupted him. Gabriel told him, "As soon as you began to pray, an answer was given, which I have come to tell you, for you are highly esteemed" (Daniel 9:23). The angel then explained what Daniel's vision would mean. At the beginning of Daniel's long prayer process, the answer was already in motion.

I suspect that this happens more often than we realize. For example, you balance your checkbook, only to find you made a mistake and now you're a little short. You pray, and in the mail that day you receive a check. The check wasn't written after you prayed. It had to have been written at least a day before. God knew your need though, and he met that specific need even before you prayed.

Sharon and I still marvel about those pre-prayer answers that came through for Crystal. God kept her and her animals safe as she walked an hour on the highway in the middle of the night. He connected her with a tow-truck driver and mechanic, who led her safely to a place to stay. The truck's problems were minimal, and she was quickly off again the next morning—so quickly that she forgot to call her mother! But the most amazing answer was the call from Hazel, the Texas college dorm mom, who could provide assurance to a very worried California mom.

God wants to answer our prayers. Sometimes all we need to do is to turn toward him and expect his amazing care for us. Just a call from us, "and the LORD will answer…and he will say: Here am I" (Isaiah 58:9).

PRAYER STARTER

Lord, thank you that you love me so much that you are ever-ready to help me when I cry out to you. Sometimes you even have already set in motion the answer to those prayers I have not even considered yet. I pray that I will be expectant as I pray—that you will welcome my words and answer in love. In Jesus' name, amen.

FITNESS TIP

If you find you're getting a side stick—a pain in your side—slow down or stop altogether for a minute or two, then begin walking again. You may be pushing it too hard, so build your intensity gradually.

Chapter 32

Conditional Answers

DAILY PRAYERWALK
Read 2 Chronicles 7:11-22.

PRAYERWALK FOCUS
"If my people, who are called by my name, will humble themselves and pray and seek my face and turn from their wicked ways, then will I hear from heaven and will forgive their sin and will heal their land."
—2 Chronicles 7:14

Before becoming a farmer, Craig had a law practice for about fifteen years. I worked for him, and during that time I learned about contracts. Essentially a contract is a binding agreement between two or more parties. The contract will spell out the obligations for each party, and if one side doesn't fulfill its obligations, the contract may be broken. We prepared contracts for people and sometimes helped them when their agreements had fallen apart. When people didn't pay what they owed us, we experienced those broken agreements firsthand and ended our relationship with them as soon as legally possible.

Sometimes God's answers to our prayers may be conditional as well. This was God's word to Solomon after he gave his sincere, long prayer of dedication for the new temple. Solomon had petitioned the Lord over and over to forgive Israel for future offenses, reminding the Lord of his contract—his covenant—with Solomon's father, David, never to fail to have a descendant of David on the throne. After the temple dedication, and after the offerings and the entire fanfare had died down and the people had gone home, the Lord answered Solomon.

This is an example that God can change his mind when we fail to uphold our end of the "prayer contract." We're familiar with the often-quoted verse "If my people, who are called by my name, will humble themselves and pray and seek my face and turn from their wicked ways, then will I hear from heaven and will forgive their sin and will heal their land" (2 Chronicles 7:14). But we're not as familiar with the statement a few verses later:

> But if you turn away and forsake the decrees and commands I have given you and go off to serve other gods and worship them, then I will uproot Israel from my land, which I have given them, and will reject this temple I have consecrated for my Name. I will make it a byword and an object of ridicule among all peoples. (verses 19-20)

God said that if they turned to him and changed their ways, he would forgive them, but if they later fell away again, his answer would change as would his favor. God says the same thing through his prophet Jeremiah (Jeremiah 18:7-10).

God's answer to Solomon's prayer was conditional. He promised that *if* the people repented and sought his face, he would hear and forgive them and heal their land of any drought or other disaster. When we look someone in the face, that person's features absorb us. We notice the eyes and nose and mouth—the whole expression. When God asks us to seek him, he wants our full attention focused on who he is, what he has said, and on what he would like. Our thoughts are full of him: We want what he wants and are ready to embrace whatever that is.

But God also said that if the people did not continue their part of the bargain, he would withdraw his favor. The conditional answer could be conditionally changed. If the people started falling away from God's laws and began following other gods, the deal was off! In fact, God said the temple would become an object of ridicule and that others would know this was a result of his people's turning from him. The crucial part of the whole contract seems to be that God required their continued faithfulness to him and him alone, and that they needed to follow his law.

God requires our faithfulness and obedience. We've seen people in public ministry fall and face ridicule. We've also seen them repent and receive God's graceful benefaction once more. The point is that God can change his answer when we change our behavior.

Just as Craig didn't have to represent clients who didn't fulfill their part of the contract, God may choose not to favor us with continued blessings when we aren't faithful anymore. As we prayerwalk, then, we'll want to seek his face and his alone—in behalf of our community, as Solomon did, and for ourselves.

Prayer Starter

Lord, each day I pray I'll know you more clearly because I've been seeking you and you alone as the One I will worship. Help me clear out anything that would distract me from that pure relationship. Teach me what it means to be humble. May I understand daily that you are God and that I am just a human, and that every breath I take should honor you. In Jesus' name, amen.

FITNESS TIP

If your shoe fits well:

1. Your longest toe won't reach the end of the shoe when you walk.
2. Your heel won't slip.
3. Your shoe won't bind the widest part of your foot.[24]

Chapter 33

When You Don't Know How to Pray

DAILY PRAYERWALK
Read Romans 8:1-27.

PRAYERWALK FOCUS
"The Spirit helps us in our weakness. We do not know what we ought to pray for, but the Spirit himself intercedes for us with groans that words cannot express."—Romans 8:26

A friend just called me. Right before midnight last night—her birthday, by the way—she learned that her father had died. He died an unhappy man: He had refused a relationship with God, spurned his family's affection, and even thrown things at his nurses. We had prayed for years that he would enter into peace with God and others, but that apparently didn't happen.

We don't have to know how to pray in order to pray; we just need to know whom to seek. Paul wrote that the Spirit helps us in our weakness:

"We do not know what we ought to pray for, but the Spirit himself intercedes for us with groans that words cannot express" (Romans 8:26). When Justin was a little guy, he swallowed a quarter. Or rather, he tried to swallow a quarter. Instead, it got stuck partway down his throat; if it had flipped, it could have stopped his breathing. We didn't know what to do, so we took him to the emergency room. After an ambulance ride to a bigger hospital and a quick surgical procedure, he was fine. We didn't know what to do, but we knew whom to call.

God knew we'd have those times when we wouldn't know how to approach him, so he gave us an intercessor through the Holy Spirit. The Greek work in Romans 8:26 for *intercede* means "to make petition or to plead on behalf of another." Someone who intercedes goes between two parties with the objective of imploring on behalf of the represented party. The Holy Spirit takes the unexpressed wishes of our heart and presents them to the Father in an earnest appeal.

The Spirit can also help us in times of despair and exhaustion. Paul wrote, "But if we hope for what we do not yet have, we wait for it patiently. In the *same way,* the Spirit helps us in our weakness" (Romans 8:25-26, emphasis added). As hope carries us through the suffering seasons of our lives, so the Spirit helps us by praying in our behalf. When you've lost someone and you're grieving, it's hard to keep track of everyday needs, such as meals—you might not even have strength to fix boxed macaroni and cheese. When someone comes to your door with supper already made, you feel comforted and helped. That's what the Spirit does for us when our heart sighs and our mind is blank. He lives in us and knows what desires lie deep within our soul and how to pray those desires according to God's will.

The Spirit can also intercede for us when we're confused and don't know how to pray. *Should I pray for healing? Should I pray my son gets one job over another? Should I pray for a new car?* God is good, and he wants his best for us, but we can't second-guess what is the ultimate good for someone else or even ourselves. In those times we can ask the Spirit to step in and intercede. And we can pray for the grace to accept God's will.

Before her father's death, my friend and I had agreed that the greatest power in prayers on behalf of her father would be the Spirit's intercession. As her father was unconscious, we had prayed that the Spirit would be interceding on this dying man's behalf. We prayed that the Spirit could accomplish in him what many on earth could not—the relating of the saving gospel in such a way that he would be convinced and drawn into the kingdom.

After his death I asked the Spirit to intercede for her family—meeting their every need in a difficult time, even at the rather confusing memorial service when the minister's words didn't match the life of my friend's father. I know those prayers were answered because I saw a new buoyancy in her following the service and in the subsequent weeks. For the rest we will just trust that God has answered as well.

I'm just a prayer pilgrim, as you may be. We need all the help we can get. With the Spirit's help, we have the hope that the Father will hear the wordless cries of our heart and will answer them in his precious way.

PRAYER STARTER

Dear Father, thank you for sending your Holy Spirit to live within me. Thank you that in those times when I'm confused or despairing or exhausted, your Spirit intercedes on my behalf. What a gift it is to know that you are hearing the desires of my heart even when I cannot express them. I pray that my heart increasingly looks more and more like yours. In Jesus' name, amen.

FITNESS TIP

Walking sticks or poles can help you remain balanced, add a little spring to your step, and give you a better workout for your arms and upper body. If you want a traditional wooden walking stick, contact Whistle Creek, the largest manufacturer of rustic walking and hiking sticks. Send three dollars for a catalog to Whistle Creek, P.O. Box 580, Monument, CO 80132, or use www.whistlecreek.com. Prices average around thirty dollars. I often use walking poles, which are available from Exerstriders, 1-800-554-0989 or www.exerstrider.com. A basic package of two poles, rubber tips, and an instructional video costs about eighty dollars. Or you can try ski poles, which are often cheap at garage sales or auctions.

Chapter 34

Waiting...and Waiting...and...

DAILY PRAYERWALK
Read Psalm 37:1-40.

PRAYERWALK FOCUS
"Be still before the LORD and wait patiently for him; do not fret when men succeed in their ways, when they carry out their wicked schemes."—Psalm 37:7

It's excruciating to wait, isn't it? You're standing in the bank line, and you know your daughter is waiting to be picked up from ball practice. Or you're on your lunch hour, you haven't even *had* lunch yet, and you're stuck at unexpected road construction on the way back from the post office, where the line went out the door.

We don't like waiting for an answer to prayer either.

I've joined my friend Maxine in waiting for God's answer to prayers for her husband and kids. As a young man he committed his life to Christ, but in recent years he hasn't attended church or read his Bible or prayed with his family. She takes the kids to church on Sunday and tries to bring them along in their own faith, but she worries that they'll wander from Christ. I ache for her and wonder myself why God hasn't answered her prayers for her husband. Wouldn't it be in God's will for John to lead his family spiritually? How many years must she wait?

The Bible doesn't answer that question directly, but it does tell us about godly people who also have had to wait. David, for example, knew the pain of waiting. Samuel anointed him king at age fifteen, but then David spent fifteen years being hunted by King Saul, who would not give up the throne. Another seven years passed before David captured Jerusalem and could move the throne there from Hebron. Eleven more years slipped by while Ammonites, Moabites, Edomites, Amalekites, and Philistines threatened almost every border. David also suffered from family problems. His older brothers resented his being favored over them, and two of his sons, Absalom and Adonijah, had power struggles with their father.[25]

We can relate to David: He had job stress, kid stress, marriage stress, and family stress. But through it all David prayed and waited. Many of the psalms are from or about David, and in Psalm 37 he gives us some insight about how to wait. Three times he uses the word *wait:* "wait patiently for Him" (verse 7, NASB) and twice "wait for the LORD" (verses 9,34, NASB).

David wrote this psalm when he was under attack, which often is the case when we're waiting for God's answer. The Enemy would have us believe that God doesn't care about us so that we turn away from him. Instead, we can do several things to ready ourselves for God's answer.

- Don't worry about those harassing you (verse 1).
- Trust in God and do good (verse 3).

- Delight in him and trust him (verses 4-5).
- Don't get angry (verse 8).

When we're waiting, it's easy to jump to a conclusion and human-reasoned action, but God's Word advises us to "Be still before the LORD and wait patiently for him" (verse 7). God wants us to quiet our zigzagging hearts and trust him. Waiting can be a good process. *The Message* says this beautifully:

> All around us we observe a pregnant creation.… That is why
> waiting does not diminish us, any more than waiting diminishes
> a pregnant mother. We are enlarged in the waiting. We, of course,
> don't see what is enlarging us. But the longer we wait, the larger we
> become, and the more joyful our expectancy. (Romans 8:22-25)

Waiting actually can grow us in Christ and make us more joyful—if we're willing.

It's hard, not being able to see around the corner, but we know that God is in control. And so Maxine waits and prays. We can wait and pray. And while we wait, we cling to God's promises from Psalm 37. He says that if we delight ourselves in him, he will give us the desires of our heart (verse 4), make our righteousness shine like the dawn and the justice of our cause like the noonday sun (verse 6), and be our stronghold in time of trouble (verse 39). And he promises that we will enjoy great peace (verse 11).

That's worth waiting for, wouldn't you agree?

PRAYER STARTER

O God of my salvation, thank you that you hear my prayers. You know it's hard to wait for answers to prayers that go over months and years because you wait so long for us to turn to you. Help me keep my eyes on your trustworthiness and your love so that I can quiet my heart and be still before you. In Jesus' name, amen.

FITNESS TIP

To challenge yourself to get in plenty of walking every day, invest in a pedometer. See if you can get in ten thousand steps a day. Pedometers are available at sports stores for twenty dollars or more.

Chapter 35

Blessing Your City

DAILY PRAYERWALK
Read Isaiah 62:1-12.

PRAYERWALK FOCUS
"For Zion's sake I will not keep silent, for Jerusalem's sake I will not remain quiet, till her righteousness shines out like the dawn, her salvation like a blazing torch."—Isaiah 62:1

In *PrayerWalk* I wrote of one morning when I felt God was giving me a vision for my small town. As I approached the city limits sign, I imagined that instead of the name of our town on the sign, it said, A Place Where God Lives. Please don't misunderstand me. It wasn't a neon daydream or a flash of heavenly light. It was more of a "what-if" moment that I believe God inspired. Right then I began praying that our town would become filled with people so transformed by God that strangers would see God's love in all of us. It's a big prayer, especially now.

I also wrote about our lumber mill, the city's only large business. When I finished *PrayerWalk,* the mill employed about 180 folks in our town of 1,200. I also wrote of my prayers for the mill workers—for their safety and spiritual transformation. These prayers, I found, were being answered. However, just before the release of *PrayerWalk,* the forests around us were closed by the government, and our mill—which had operated for about one hundred years—also closed. Suddenly men who had worked their entire adult lives in that plant were out of work, putting together résumés for the first time, and seeking jobs in the city, an hour away.

Sadly, some folks began to give our town a virtual death sentence. The *Los Angeles Times*'s headline read: "Sierra Sawmill's Closing Leaves a Town and Its Workers Grasping for a Future." The article quoted a California Forestry Association spokesman who said our town would "be hurt. This will have a huge ripple effect." Expecting declining enrollments in our town's schools, the school district sent layoff notices for teachers. Even the students seemed to agree. "It'll be a ghost town," one said in our high school newspaper.

The negativity was beginning to affect me as well, until I read a verse I am claiming for our town: "When right-living people bless the city, it flourishes; evil talk turns it into a ghost town in no time" (Proverbs 11:11, MSG). I typed up this verse, framed it, and pray that God will bless our city.

Isaiah also wouldn't quit praying for his city. He wrote that he wouldn't keep silent until Jerusalem shone "like the dawn," "like a blazing torch" (62:1). He also called her other beautiful, metaphorical names—"crown of splendor," "a royal diadem" (verse 3)—and wanted God to rejoice over the city as a bridegroom delights in his new bride (verse 5). He even posted watchmen to pray day and night for Jerusalem and urged all who called on God to pray continually until God made Jerusalem "the praise of the earth" (verse 7).

Can you imagine your town being the "praise of the earth"—a city so beautiful in God's sight that it would be given a new name? Isaiah had that hope for Jerusalem and spoke of several new names throughout his book that God would place upon his city:

- City of Righteousness (Isaiah 1:26)
- Faithful City (Isaiah 1:26)
- The City of the LORD (Isaiah 60:14)
- Zion of the Holy One of Israel (Isaiah 60:14)
- The Holy People (Isaiah 62:12)
- The Redeemed of the LORD (Isaiah 62:12)
- Sought After (Isaiah 62:12)
- The City No Longer Deserted (Isaiah 62:12)

I was particularly struck, though, when I read of the name God gave Ezekiel for the future Jerusalem, because it was so similar to the one I felt God had given me for my town. After listing the exact measurements of the gates of the new, restored Jerusalem, Ezekiel wrote, "And the name of the city from that time on will be: THE LORD IS THERE" (Ezekiel 48:35). *A place where God lives...the Lord is there...* wouldn't it be wonderful to be able to say either phrase about our communities?

As I write this, our town's hardship pales in the light of the devastation in New York City following the destruction of the World Trade Center towers. But even in the shadows of loss, God's light can shine in the lives of his people. Most of our townspeople gathered on our Main Street to pray for the victims to seek God's forgiveness, grace, and blessing for all of us. I refuse to believe that tragedy, loss, and evil will reign. God has his hand on our communities, and we can become "a place where God lives."

Be an Isaiah or an Ezekiel for your town. For its sake do not keep silent in prayer—call on God night and day until your community is a blazing torch, guiding others to our loving Savior.

PRAYER STARTER

Dear Lord, I ask you to bless my community greatly. Make it a city on a hill—so beautiful and desirable in your eyes that others are drawn to it to beg the question: "What makes this place different?" May each person choose you as the Savior of their lives and choose a Spirit-filled day-to-day difference so that other communities are changed as well. In Jesus' name, amen.

FITNESS TIP

To avoid back problems from walking incorrectly, keep your rear end tucked underneath you, tightening your stomach muscles. Check your posture before you leave your home by standing against a wall and flattening your stomach.[26]

Chapter 36

When You Can Do More Than Pray

DAILY PRAYERWALK
Read Luke 10:1-24.

PRAYERWALK FOCUS
"When you enter a house, first say, 'Peace to this house.'"—Luke 10:5

Prayer for those in need is critical, but sometimes we can do even more. We can help meet the tangible needs of those for whom we pray. That tangible help could be a meal, housecleaning help, a drive to the doctor's office, or a financial gift. It could be helping a friend clean up her flooded home. It could also mean donating sick days to a fellow employee.

A praying friend, Sue, has been an effective leader against the hold of poverty in my town. A couple of years ago she realized she had no need for the large workshop on her property in the middle of town and sensed that God was calling her to start a community food bank. She began the ministry through our church, and with the encouragement and support of county social services personnel, she has pretty much single-handedly carried it all these months. Our town is not a rich town, and homes are very simple. Even when the lumber mill closed earlier this year and half the adult male population became unemployed, poverty could not get a grip on our town because of Sue's food bank and the other generous folks who'd deliver a free load of wood or provide a ride or a meal. Our town is bouncing back, even though life looked pretty bleak for a time. Many are not only praying but also caring tangibly for others.

Luke tells us that when Jesus appointed two-man teams to go into the towns where he later planned to teach and preach, he instructed them in etiquette and told them to do four things: to pray, to bless, to heal, and to say, "The kingdom of God is near" (Luke 10:11).

By praying, we are helping to heal the cracks of others' lives; in effect we are taking the kingdom of God to the people in our neighborhood or job or community at large. After we pray, we can extend our prayerwalk through acts of caring that will help others see Christ in us and perhaps even draw them closer to God. In *Taking Our Cities for God*, John Dawson says that this overcoming evil with good is one form of spiritual warfare. One simple example of this might be supporting those businesses you pray for—by shopping there. What good does it do that merchant in your neighborhood if you pray for him regularly but buy elsewhere? This can encourage him and provide healing if he is suffering financially. Establishing a relationship in this way first provides a natural opportunity later to speak of the love of Christ.

One dear friend and her husband have a small appliance store in my town. I pray that God will bless their business. I ask her regularly what prayer needs she might have and pray for those as well. Instead of buying my appliances at a discount store in Reno, I shop at my friends' store. I figure that I am helping fulfill my own prayer that God bless their business. I also recommend their products without qualification and joke about the time when I rushed into the store one day, announcing, "I need to buy a dryer, and I've only got ten minutes!" A half-hour later the new one was installed in my house!

Jesus taught that our prayer life is esse tial, but he also taught that we should help meet each other's physical .ieeds. We take the kingdom of God to one another by preparing with prayer, caring in tangible ways, and then sharing that we're doing it in the name of Jesus.

Prayer Starter

Father, remind me that my ministry does not end with prayer, but that I can also help meet the needs of my neighbors and friends in simple ways. Give me the empathy and boldness you demonstrated to your disciples. Thank you for the privilege of taking your kingdom to my community. In Jesus' name, amen.

Fitness Tip

You can help extend the life of your walking shoes by

- machine-washing them in a short cycle using warm or cold water,
- using sandpaper to rough up worn sole areas,
- applying two layers of a shoe-patching product on the entire sole,
- replacing the insole with a store-bought insert.[27]

Chapter 37

Praying for Your Enemies

DAILY PRAYERWALK
Read Matthew 5:43-48.

PRAYERWALK FOCUS
"Love your enemies and pray for those who persecute you."
—Matthew 5:44

My friend Maxine finds that one of the first pickup trucks she passes while prayerwalking each morning is Tom's. She waves; he nods. They used to look the other way and pretend they hadn't seen each other. He'd shift in his seat behind the wheel. She'd hum "Nearer My God to Thee" or something. The thing was she wasn't nearer her God at that moment, because she wasn't following Jesus' words to love and pray for her enemies.

Tom and her husband were once business partners. They had a falling out and divided up the various assets of the partnership. Tom then sued both her husband and Maxine. She never understood how she was part of any of it. She was just a wife trying to be a good mom. But she found herself answering questions at depositions and facing Tom and his wife across a table more than once, praying that God would just end the whole thing so that she wouldn't get stomachaches anymore.

Jesus taught, though, that we must go the extra mile past the written, scriptural law. He said:

- He had come not to abolish the law but to fulfill it (Matthew 5:17).
- An insult is just as wrong as murder (Matthew 5:22).
- Though the law would permit retribution, I should turn the other cheek (Matthew 5:39).
- If someone would sue me for my dress, I should also give him my coat (Matthew 5:40).

In biblical times a passerby might be pressed into military service and forced to travel with a company, perhaps even carrying some equipment. This was true for Simon, who was enlisted to carry the cross when Jesus' strength gave out. Jesus instructs that if "someone forces you to go one mile, go with him two miles" (Matthew 5:41). In other words, the requirement of the law is never enough. As believers we must do more than the bottom line. I smile and think of that passage sometimes when I talk my prayerwalking partners into going one more mile of the valley road.

I've benefited many times from friends who've gone the extra mile with me. Diana rode with me in a Ryder rental truck all the way from Kansas, caring for twenty-month-old Rebekah and six-month-old Justin while I followed Craig to California along Interstate 80. She not only bounced along and cared for my babies, but she also put up with Craig's and my sharp words every time we pulled into a stopping spot. Joyce manned our law office fort while I went back to school to get my teaching credentials, and she also watched Joshua, then a preschooler. I must owe my friend June a hundred dinners for all the times she has left hot food on my kitchen counter when she knew I'd been having hard school days.

We'll do nearly anything for a friend too, but how about going the extra mile for someone who doesn't like us? That doesn't even make sense! But God doesn't operate according to human wisdom, and when we obey him when things don't make sense, we give him glory.

One morning when Maxine was talking with God about why he hadn't ended the lawsuit, Tom drove by. He shifted in his seat as usual, she pretended she didn't see him, and he accelerated down the highway out of town. But as she watched him make the bend of the road that morning, she felt something different. There was no magical *aha!* Just a pull from God to pray *for* Tom—not just for the *case* but for the *man.*

She began to ask God to bless him and his marriage and his family and his business. She prayed that way every time she saw him, and within two weeks the lawsuit that had plagued their lives for four years was settled. When she stopped praying for the case and started praying for the man, the ugly mess suddenly ended. A short time later she ran into his wife at a local restaurant, hugged her, and oohed and aahed over her new grandchild.

Who knows what miracle moments like that we can all have when we begin praying for our enemies.

PRAYER STARTER

Dear Father, forgive me for holding back prayer for ones who've caused me pain. I ask you to bless them today. Thank you, Lord, that your warming sun and refreshing rain fall over us all to remind us that you love us equally. In Jesus' name, amen.

FITNESS TIP

Watch your step on rainy days. Avoid puddles, white road stripes, and mossy areas. Wear bright clothing, garments that breathe, and shoes with rippled soles.

Chapter 38

Partners with God

DAILY PRAYERWALK
Read Isaiah 6.

PRAYERWALK FOCUS
"Then I heard the voice of the Lord saying, 'Whom shall I send? And who will go for us?' And I said, 'Here am I. Send me!'"—Isaiah 6:8

After I became a Christian, I finished my journalism degree, married Craig, and headed out into the work world. When he was stationed with the army in Kansas, I pounded the streets as a newspaper reporter and served as religion editor. Even though I was writing about God, I didn't feel that God had *called* me to write about him.[28] I was just doing a job.

That all changed one summer fifteen years ago when I went off with friends to a women's retreat in the Sierras south of beautiful Lake Tahoe. The retreat speaker had told us to go off somewhere by ourselves into the woods and sit until God spoke to us. I found a large rock under some pine trees and started praying. All of a sudden I stopped and simply looked around me. The hundred-foot Ponderosa pines seemingly created a cathedral right before my eyes. The sun's rays directed my eyes toward the spotlessly blue sky. The wind seemed to whisper praise, and I was struck with the incredible magnificence of all that God had created in that one little spot of heaven on earth.

Then I heard him: "I want you to write for me." The words weren't in the wind but deep inside me.

The sensation was so clear, so direct, that I remember standing and saying aloud, "How, Lord?" I didn't get explicit direction that day, but two weeks later I did, at a writers' conference in Minneapolis. I've been writing out of a sense of calling ever since. The call I heard that day years ago changed my life. I live my days with purpose as I put words on paper and pray that others find encouragement from them.

Isaiah's life was also changed by God's call. At the time of his call, the king he had been serving, Uzziah, had just died, and as a priest, Isaiah was probably busy at work in the temple. The temple wasn't like our church today. In fact, the two Old Testament, Hebrew words for temple—*bayit* and *hikhal*—mean "house of God" and "Yahweh's palace." The Jews saw the temple as the resting place for God, and the priests were very busy at work in his house.

When God came to him, Isaiah could have been burning an animal's suet or kidneys on the altar. He may have been sprinkling ewe's blood on the altar's horns or boiling a cereal offering. Or he may have just been cleaning house. In any case, Isaiah apparently was alone when the Lord revealed himself—seated on a throne, the hem of his robe so large that it filled the temple. The angels' music was greater than a rock concert. Doorposts and thresholds shook, and REAL smoke filled the temple.

When Isaiah heard the voice of the Lord, "Whom shall I send? And who will go for us?" he responded, "Here am I. Send me!" (Isaiah 6:8). From those five little "yes" words, Isaiah went on to prophesy for about sixty years under the reigns of Jotham, Ahaz, and Hezekiah. Many consider him the greatest of the writing prophets.

God can call us to do more than one thing for him, and after I'd been prayerwalking for a couple of months, God also called me to intercede for my town. Instead of praying sporadically for the needs in my town, I knew God had chosen me to pray on a daily basis for those in my community. As I now walk up and down the main street of my town, I ask that he will bless our businesses, heal the hurts, and bring us together as a godly people. My words, whether on paper or in prayer, aren't inspired poetry or prose like Isaiah's, but neither are they the product of a job. God's graceful calls have changed me from someone doing a job to someone working alongside him.

Is God calling you to partner with him in ministry? Listen for his clear voice as you seek him today.

PRAYER STARTER

Dear Lord, here I am. Some days it doesn't seem as though I have much to offer. I have no fancy words for my prayers. Some days I'm just plodding along, one foot in front of the other. But I'm willing to pray and to listen for your direction. Open my ears to your call and my heart to the prayer needs around me. Here I am! Send me! In Jesus' name, amen!

FITNESS TIP

On a hot day drink water an hour or so before your walk to avoid dehydration. Your bladder will probably empty before you head out.

Chapter 39

Rending Your Heart

Read Joel 2:1-13.

PRAYERWALK FOCUS

"Rend your heart and not your garments. Return to the LORD your God, for he is gracious and compassionate, slow to anger and abounding in love, and he relents from sending calamity."—Joel 2:13

My heart has broken many times as my town has gone through great difficulties. Four times in just the last twenty years floods have swept through it. Craig and our kids and I had not been in our new house even one year when the first flood crept up to our doorsill. A year later the water was several inches deep throughout our first floor. Later that year we had our house raised four and a half feet. Since then floods have twice invaded our neighbors' homes and closed roads and schools. Then came the forest fire. We live at the edge of a national forest in a beautiful mountain valley. Eight years ago four major news networks covered the Cottonwood fire that threatened our town several times and burned over forty-eight thousand acres of beautiful trees. The size of our town tripled for a week while firefighters from all across the country stood the lines around our town. Last year drought plagued local farmers and ranchers, with the president declaring our county eligible for national assistance.

Maybe that's why I can relate so well to the pain on the pages of the book of Joel. The few short chapters from the prophet of Jerusalem speak of a three-pronged devastation. Wave after wave of locust swarms—generations of them, young and old—ate their way through the harvest fields. They moved so strongly that the locusts were compared to a mighty army, galloping along like cavalry with a noise like chariots'.

But they were only the first assault. Drought was the locusts' companion. Seeds shriveled beneath the clods of dirt. Granaries fell down. Cattle moaned. Then fire licked up what those greedy forces left behind. Vines were stripped. Fig trees withered. The priests mourned because there was nothing for the daily grain or drink offerings. Joel wrote the Lord's words: "Surely the joy of mankind is withered away" (1:12).

Joel called the people together solely for the purpose of seeking repentance. He said, "Put on sackcloth, O priests, and mourn" (1:13). Sackcloth was an itchy material taken from grain bags. The itch would not let them put the pain behind. People would rend or tear their sackcloth garments in moments of emotional repentance or national mourning. Joel also told the priests, "Declare a holy fast; call a sacred assembly. Summon the elders and all who live in the land to the house of the LORD your God, and cry out to the LORD" (1:14).

But God wanted more than outward gestures that the people were turning to him. "'Even now,' declares the LORD, 'return to me with all your heart, with fasting and weeping'" (2:12). Joel told the people that God wanted torn hearts, hearts broken up and shredded by the thought that they would try to manage their lives without him.

I don't know if the disasters that have come to my town are the results of God's judgment, like the swarm of locusts upon Jerusalem. Maybe they are; maybe they aren't. That really isn't important—what matters is what such disasters reveal about my heart. Is my trust in God alone? Do I live in the awareness of my utter dependence upon him?

This can be hard when we face hardship, and we tend to muster all our wits to try to figure our way through the mire. We want to do something to solve the problem. Instead, we must first go to God.

Now my town faces economical disaster from the mill's closing, and my heart hurts as I prayerwalk. I had considered the commuting mill workers and the loggers my friends. I pray for them still. I'm asking that God will provide jobs that allow them to keep their children in our good schools—that those jobs will be even better ones than before. I'm asking that the stress of being unemployed not break down families and that each person will turn to God for his or her strength.

When disaster strikes, you and I can join together as the people did with Joel—each in our own towns, but each with a common mission: to offer up prayers for those who are suffering from the devastation that seems often to accompany life in this world. "Rend" your heart as Joel did and pray—and just see what God will do.

PRAYER STARTER

Father, I'd like to be able to see—maybe just a glimpse—how your heart breaks for my town. Do you weep when teenagers tell their parents they don't want to go to church anymore? Or when a father decides he doesn't love the mother of his children…and leaves? Or when your people give lip service on Sunday and then slip into the crowd at work the next day? Show me how to pray, Lord, for the hurting, the lost, and the indifferent. Give me the courage to give my heart over in prayer to you. In Jesus' name, amen.

FITNESS TIP

If your feet or joints begin to hurt after you've been walking for a few months, consider getting new shoes. The tread or the inner support may be worn down and may not be cushioning your foot as it should. You'll need a new pair at least every five hundred miles of walking, maybe sooner if you wear your shoes for anything other than walking. I replace mine every four to six months.

Chapter 40

No Lone Wolves

DAILY PRAYERWALK
Read Acts 2:42-47.

PRAYERWALK FOCUS
"They devoted themselves to the apostles' teaching and to the fellowship, to the breaking of bread and to prayer."—Acts 2:42

A year or so after I started prayerwalking, I began to think of certain people and situations as my prayer babies and of prayerwalking as "my" ministry. I was silently claiming ownership over the areas where I prayerwalked. One day when a friend said she also was walking and praying along Main Street, I suggested that maybe she'd want to prayerwalk somewhere else in town. I remember saying something like, "I've got it covered."

She looked me straight in the eye and said, "Janet, I'd like to pray for these people too."

Prayer can be a lonely occupation, and it's possible for a prayerwalker or other intercessor to feel a little territorial or even self-righteous if she or he is isolated from other Christians. Consistent fellowship can remind us that we are part of a larger ministry, of something far greater that God is doing in the world.

In Acts we're told that the believers "devoted themselves to the apostles' teaching and to the fellowship, to the breaking of bread and to prayer" (2:42). They studied the Bible together, worshiped together, and prayed together. Doing so much in concert with each other would have allowed time for teaching, questioning, correcting, and encouraging.

This balance of prayer, worship, fellowship, and study is essential for the community of believers. For one thing, we need the encouragement and support of other Christians. This reminds us that we are not the only ones who love God and try to represent him in this world. Other Christians can also stimulate our faith and strengthen us during those times when we feel discouraged. Another reason we need fellowship is that other believers can hold us accountable. For instance, if I return to church after being gone a week, folks will ask, "Where were you last week?" That's healthy for me—to know that others are watching out for my spiritual well-being. It's also healthy to hear my pastor preach the Word and to hear others discuss it.

Some might feel a little prayer here and a verse there is enough. However, Hebrews 10:25 says, "Let us not give up meeting together, as some are in the habit of doing, but let us encourage one another—and all the more as you see the Day approaching." If the early Christians needed each other's teaching and encouragement, surely we must as well. When we're alone, we're easier prey for the Enemy and his darts of discouragement, doubt, despair, or deception—which can, in turn, get our prayers off track.

Each of us helps make up the Christian body; when we don't worship and pray and serve with our local church, the body does not function as well. Each of us is needed—in fact, each of us is indispensable (1 Corinthians 12:22). I might not need encouragement on a particular Sunday, but I might be the only one who would notice that Margaret does. If I'm not there, who'll be my eyes, ears, and voice for her? My church needs me to use my gifts, and it needs me to be part of its praying body.

Leadership especially needs prayerwalkers in the pews. John Maxwell writes in *Partners in Prayer* that many pastors "are discouraged and ready to quit the ministry. And many times the people in their church aren't aware of the struggles they're going through."[29] Our spiritual leaders need our prayers, support, and caring.

Will that church experience be perfect? No. We all need prayer. Some Sundays I just sit in our sanctuary and put on my prayerwalk eyes—praying for individuals in the pews and those leading worship. You can take your praying heart and join with me in church this Sunday. No lone wolf howling allowed.

PRAYER STARTER

Father, thank you that I don't have to be a lone wolf in prayer and that your Son created a model for community with his seeking out of the twelve disciples. Thank you for the larger Christian body, and that I've been given gifts that are crucial to its functioning well—even my intercession for others. Keep me in fellowship—for the benefit of the body and for the benefit of my own healthy spiritual growth. In Jesus' name, amen.

FITNESS TIP

If you like walking with a group and plan to go on vacation, you can check out Volksmarches. There are over nineteen hundred of these events in the U.S.—special walks through historical or other interesting areas. The shortest walk will be a 10-kilometer (6.2-mile) walk. You can call the American Volkssport Association for information at (210) 659-2112, 1-800-830-WALK, or AVAHQ@aol.com.

Chapter 41

In God We Trust

PRAYERWALK FOCUS
"My Father, if it is not possible for this cup to be taken away unless I drink it, may your will be done."—Matthew 26:42

During my friend Rose's ten-year battle with cancer, many people prayed for her. Because she was on radio and television, hundreds, maybe thousands, of Christians prayed faithfully that God would heal her. We would read the New Testament verses on healing over and over and think: *God could heal Rose.* Some felt Rose would be healed and even told her so, confident that healing was God's will for her. Yet we watched her decline, first slowly, then quickly.

Eventually I found peace praying both for Rose's healing and for God's will. I could pray in faith for healing because I knew my Creator and Sustainer was big enough and great enough to heal anyone of anything. I also prayed for his will for Rose because I could not know his plan for her.

Rose lost the battle with cancer but gained the kingdom of God.

As I grappled with God over Rose's death, I gained comfort and understanding from the prayers Jesus prayed just before his death. I would venture to say that every earthly onlooker at Calvary would have thought Christ had lost the battle. Even his last words indicate a giving up:

"Father, forgive them, for they do not know what they are doing." (Luke 23:34)

"My God, my God, why have you forsaken me?" (Matthew 27:46; also Mark 15:34)

"Father, into your hands I commit my spirit." (Luke 23:46)

The self-proclaimed messiah was dead. The one who healed and taught and fed thousands both literally and figuratively was dead. The carpenter who dared to question the intent of the law was dead. His persecutors had won. Or so it seemed.

But the truth is, Jesus' prayers were answered. Earlier in the evening he had prayed:

"My father, if it is possible, may this cup be taken from me. Yet not as I will, but as you will." (Matthew 26:39; also see Mark 14:36 and Luke 22:42)

"My Father, if it is not possible for this cup to be taken away unless I drink it, may your will be done." (Matthew 26:42)

Jesus prayed what he as a man, a mother's son, wanted, but he also prayed for what his heavenly Father would want. He asked that if there were another way, that he not have to face the suffering of the cross, but he also prayed that his Father's will would be done.

It's a dichotomy of prayer, I think, to lay before God what we want and then sincerely request that God's will be done. It's an honest, human prayer. It's also a good, heaven-seeking prayer. In the process of the prayer—the actual words as they're thought and realized and accepted and said—the pray-er becomes an instrument of God's will. When we seek his will, we grow into and become that will. Herbert Lockyer said it well: "The whole purpose of prayer is the accomplishment of His known will."[30] My prayers are my best human attempt at a holy act—if only in the seeking of his perfect will.

Prayer isn't a formula. I can't take God's will, plus a right attitude and a clean conscience and a perfect motive and know I'll get the answer I want. The answer is *God's* decision, and he alone knows what is best. So I pray "thy will be done" and allow God to let me ride on the edge of his daily grace, which is sufficient for me. God takes my prayers and works his will with us humans who often willfully do not follow him. That's the miracle. His perfect will is worked through imperfect me—and you.

PRAYER STARTER

Oh, Father, even though I read your Word and wait for your voice, sometimes I just don't know what you would have for others or me. Help me pray in your will, Lord. Take me to the place where everything I desire is only that which is completely centered in you. Make me a vessel that can only hold that which is pleasing in your sight. In Jesus' name, amen.

FITNESS TIP

It's hard to stay motivated. Here are several tips to get out the door offered in *The 90-Day Fitness Walking Program:*

- Put on your walking clothes. This will help you anticipate the workout.
- Tell others you're going. They'll remind you of your commitment.
- Work for a streak. When I started, I kept track of how many days in a row I had walked. Try for one hundred straight days, even if some of your walks are more like strolls.[31]

Chapter 42

Going Deeper

DAILY PRAYERWALK

Read Isaiah 58:1-14.

PRAYERWALK FOCUS

"Your fasting ends in quarreling and strife, and in striking each other with wicked fists. You cannot fast as you do today and expect your voice to be heard on high."—Isaiah 58:4

For a period of time I fasted on Wednesdays to focus more on God in regard to important personal and family needs. Craig was in graduate school, working toward an advanced degree that could lead to teaching at the college level, and I was considering taking a leave from teaching for a half year or longer. I wanted God's guidance regarding these decisions: I wanted them hemmed in by prayer.

I'm a Janet-come-lately to fasting. Because I have struggled with dieting and bulimia, I had been counseled in the past not to fast out of concern that I might enter into it with the wrong motives. I might be more focused on the control issues than on the central purpose of fast-

ing—"a means by which we can worship the Lord and submit ourselves in humility to Him."[32]

So I decided to study about fasting in order to be sure it was right
for me at this juncture in my life. I read a very helpful book, *Fasting for
Spiritual Breakthrough* by Elmer L. Towns, from which I learned that
biblical folks fasted with various objectives: to solve problems, to pray
for revival, to break fears, and so on.

I also researched what God's Word has to say about fasting. While
the Bible doesn't command us to fast, Jesus seemed to imply that we
will when he said, "*When* you fast…" (Matthew 6:16, emphasis added).
In that passage he teaches that fasting should be done privately, without
drawing attention to yourself or what you're doing. In Isaiah 58 we
learn that those who fast are hypocritical if their wrong behavior doesn't
change. Fasting should move us to better behavior—helping those in
need, for example. If we don't see this kind of change in our lives, God
says, "You cannot fast as you do today and expect your voice to be
heard on high" (Isaiah 58:4).

Fasting, then, is centered on God, not self. Richard Foster writes,
"It must be God-initiated and God-ordained."[33] We don't fast because
we want to get something out of God or because we're spiritualizing a
weight-loss program. We fast to grow toward complete dependence on
God. Dallas Willard says that in fasting "we learn by experience that
God's word to us is a life substance, that it is not food ("bread") alone
that gives life, but also the words that proceed from the mouth of God
(Matthew 4:4)."[34]

As I reflected on my motives, I decided to fast. I've never been dis-
appointed when I've earnestly sought God for guidance. God called me
to write after a deeper time in prayer. While I waited for his direction
for those life changes, I found that God took me deeper into my relationship with him.

If you decide to fast, you might want to use the following steps outlined by Bill Bright:[35]

- Set an objective. For what purpose do you want to fast and pray?
- Make a commitment. What kind of fast would you undertake? No solid food? Restricted solid food? Only water? Drink enough water; many drink fruit juice.
- Prepare yourself spiritually. Do you sincerely want more of God's influence? If not, confess those things that stand in the way.
- Prepare yourself physically. Eat lightly two days before the fast. Consult your doctor if you are on medication or have any ailment, such as diabetes, that would be influenced by a fast.
- Set a schedule. How will you fill the time you'd otherwise be preparing and eating food? Perhaps others could support your fast joyfully by fixing their meals on that day. Then you can read the Bible, pray, or sing to the Lord.
- End your fast gradually, so you don't traumatize your body.

We can expect results to our prayers when we fast. God even promises to bless us: "Then you will find your joy in the LORD, and I will cause you to ride on the heights of the land and to feast on the inheritance of your father Jacob" (Isaiah 58:14).

Isn't that just like our God? We fast and God promises a feast. We give up a little, and he showers us with even more than we would have had.

PRAYER STARTER

Lord, I realize that I am completely dependent upon you in this world. I desire to grow closer to you and to know you more deeply through fasting. Help me examine my heart to see if there be any wrong motive as I seek you in this way. Give me the discipline and strength to follow through—and the excited expectancy to wait for the results in my life. Draw me closer in whatever way you would choose. In Jesus' name, amen.

FITNESS TIP

Do not deprive yourself of liquids when you exercise. If your bladder can tolerate water intake while you walk, you might want to consider investing in a water reservoir device. Good sporting goods stores carry these liquid pouches. You strap the twenty- to ninety-ounce holder onto your back and thread a long, pliable straw through your clothing so that the straw reaches your mouth. Then you can sip as you desire. They cost thirty dollars or more.

Chapter 43

From Heaven to Earth

DAILY PRAYERWALK
Read Ephesians 6:10-20.

PRAYERWALK FOCUS
"And pray in the Spirit on all occasions with all kinds of prayers and requests. With this in mind, be alert and always keep on praying for all the saints."—Ephesians 6:18

I met a woman named Ann the other day at a convention. She and I chatted for a while about prayerwalking when I noticed a heaviness in her spirit. I asked if she had a prayer need, and she started crying, saying that her business was failing because of new competition surrounding her. She felt attacked by the Enemy, and she didn't know if she should keep the business. After I prayed against the spirit of discouragement, I asked God to come alongside and encourage her. We shared a hug and that prayer, and she seemed to lighten a bit just knowing, I think, that someone else cared.

In our walk as pray-ers, we will sometimes be faced with situations when we sense the Enemy's influence. If Satan dared to tempt even Jesus, how much more will he try to make us falter? I do not tiptoe through my life looking for Satan behind every door, but I know that he tries to sidetrack believers through discouragement, deception, doubt, or despair. When I was talking with Ann, God gave me the discernment to point out that she wasn't seeing things from his perspective but was only looking at the numbers in her accounting book. When I prayed, I spoke directly to the spirits of discouragement and deception and commanded them to leave her alone. Instantly I felt the tenseness leave her body, and her eyes showed a spark I hadn't seen before.

Richard Foster calls this a prayer of command or authoritative prayer.[36] He says that normally we pray earth to heaven. With authoritative prayer, we're using the authority given us by Christ (Ephesians 2:6) and praying heaven to earth. Just as Jesus spoke simple commands such as the one that calmed the sea, so can we pray a prayer of command to still the raging waters of emotions or illness or pain. I personally have seen my fears disappear, my children's worries fade, and physical pain in my body evaporate when I have prayed authoritatively.

Christians are exhorted not to be passive in the battle against Satan. In the well-known passage in Ephesians 6 about the armor of God, Paul admonishes us not to allow ourselves to become casualties, but instead to stand against the devil's schemes. He goes on to tell us to put on the armor of God. That armor includes:

- Truth. Instead of gossiping or deceiving, we speak the truth in love.
- Righteousness. We do what's right. Instead of allowing even shades of racial intolerance in our neighborhoods or schools or workplaces, we become bridges, a people willing to erase completely the lines that divide us.

- Readiness. When God calls us to a task—whether it's a church committee or a position on our local school board—we step forward immediately.
- The gospel of peace. We tear down the fences of our relationships and do it all as a testimony to the life of Jesus Christ, which we freely share.
- Faith. We believe that God is trustworthy, and we live fearlessly for Christ.
- Salvation. We recognize that we are saved by the gracious gift of our Lord, not of anything that we have done, and we extend that grace to others so that they are drawn to eternity as well.
- The Bible. We study God's Word and use it to guide our speech and actions.
- Prayer. Paul tells us to pray *four times:* "Pray in the spirit on all occasions" (verse 18), "be alert and always keep on praying" (verse 18), "Pray also for me" (verse 19), and "Pray that I may declare it [the gospel] fearlessly" (verse 20). Prayer is a great weapon, especially when used with the other armor God has given us.

When these "weapons" are used together—when we have faith, have studied God's Word, and live out our life in a way that glorifies him—the Enemy has a strong contender.

About a half-hour after my meeting with Ann, I finished with my meetings and headed for the ladies' room. Guess who was there? Ann. "Oh," she said, "I had just prayed I'd run into you again. I wanted to let you know that I feel so much better. The burdens seem to have lifted."

PRAYER STARTER
Thank you, Father, that you did not leave your children defenseless here on earth but gave us your Holy Spirit and many spiritual weapons.

Thank you for extending the authority you gave your Son also to us so we can stand against the Enemy's schemes. Keep me close to you so that my testimony stays clean and strong. Help me bind your Word to my heart, ever ready in times of trouble. In Jesus' name, amen.

FITNESS TIP

Fitness Walking for Dummies offers several safety tips, including:

- Walk defensively.
- Make sure someone at home knows your route.
- Keep the volume low on your headset, so you can hear someone approaching.
- Be alert in wooded or brushy areas.
- Consider carrying mace or a police whistle.
- Take a partner or go to the mall.[37]

Chapter 44

Stamp of Approval

DAILY PRAYERWALK
Read Haggai 2:1-23.

PRAYERWALK FOCUS
"'I will make you like my signet ring, for I have chosen you,' declares the LORD Almighty."—Haggai 2:23

In the short book of Haggai, God speaks to Zerubbabel through the prophet Haggai. Zerubbabel[38] was named governor of Judah by Cyrus, the Persian king who allowed the Jews to return to Jerusalem. Although Cyrus gave Zerubbabel the task of leading the state, God had an additional job in mind—rebuilding the temple for the Jews who had returned from exile in Babylon.

God told Zerubbabel that he would make Zerubbabel like his signet ring, "for I have chosen you" (Haggai 2:23). A signet ring had a design worked into the stone or metal that represented its owner and wearer, the king, and was used to indicate royal authority. The ring would be pushed into the warm wax that sealed the document requiring the king's mark. God was signaling that Zerubbabel was God's mark or representative—his seal—in Jerusalem.

The Bible uses seals in several ways, but in each case the seal of the signet ring is the sign of its owner: It symbolizes authority, witness, and security. The pharaoh gave his seal to Joseph to indicate the authority passing to his new second in command (Genesis 41:42). Jeremiah sealed his deed to land bought from his cousin to indicate a witness of the signature (Jeremiah 32:10). A seal could keep something secure, such as the unrevealed prophecy in Daniel 12:9 and the scroll in Revelation 5:1.

When God chose Zerubbabel and gave him his signet ring, God was putting his authority on Zerubbabel. The earthly king would be the representative for his heavenly King.

God has also chosen us and given us a seal. Paul tells us that when we believed, we were "marked in him with a seal, the promised Holy Spirit, who is a deposit guaranteeing our inheritance until the redemption of those who are in God's possession" (Ephesians 1:13-14). We have God's stamp of approval.

As God's representative on earth, I believe I have the special privilege and responsibility to stand before God in my community and to pray for its needs. Because I have the Holy Spirit within me, I can see the people of my town through God's eyes. I see a man struggling to get to work with his falling-apart pickup and pray for that family's finances. I see a loaded logging truck *leaving* the lumber mill and pray for the men who have lost jobs because of our mill's recent permanent closure. I hear a business owner lose his cool in the early morning hours and pray for peace in that family and that company.

Andrew Murray agrees that interceding for others is a privilege. In one of his last chapters in *The Ministry of Intercessory Prayer,* he writes nine times: "God needs intercessors" and includes the observation from Isaiah: "And he saw that there was no man, and wondered that there was no intercessor" (Isaiah 59:16, KJV).

Maybe you're also being called for this great privilege. Perhaps you can wear the signet ring of the King in your community. Go ahead. Put it on and walk in the security that God has given you. Be his witness. Ask for his eyesight for your community and then pray with his authority.

PRAYER STARTER
Thank you, Father, that you have sealed me as your own. May I wear your mark with boldness, sensitivity, and honor. May I make a difference in the lives of those who live and work around me. Grace me with your eyesight, Lord, so that I can pray with clarity and conviction. May others, in turn, then also wear your signet ring. In Jesus' name, amen.

FITNESS TIP
Ladies only: If you don't feel your sports bra is supporting you as much as you need, try wearing your regular bra underneath. If that's not comfortable, try wearing an encapsulation sports bra underneath a compression sports bra.

Chapter 45

Finding Sanctuary

DAILY PRAYERWALK
Read Ezekiel 11:16-25.

PRAYERWALK FOCUS
"Therefore say: 'This is what the Sovereign LORD says: Although I sent them far away among the nations and scattered them among the countries, yet for a little while I have been a sanctuary for them in the countries where they have gone.'"—Ezekiel 11:16

Often we go to prayer because we need a safe, quiet place. Our private worlds may be, at best, crowded with activity and a little chaotic, at worst threatening. There are times when I'm figuratively running to prayer—when I'm overwhelmed by the gloom of newspaper headlines, by a rush of demands from family and work, or even by unkind remarks from an upset student or parent. In prayer God becomes my sanctuary.

The Jews understood this need for a safe place. God had given them the Promised Land, and the walls of Jerusalem symbolized God's care and protection of them as a people. But when Jerusalem was captured, forcing the Jews into exile in Babylon, this sense of sanctuary was stripped from them. Through the prophet Ezekiel, God told the people, "Although I sent them far away among the nations and scattered them among the countries, yet for a little while I have been a sanctuary for them in the countries where they have gone" (Ezekiel 11:16). Even though the Jewish nation was in a foreign land, the Jews still could be at home there as their Lord was with them.

Scripture reminds us that God can be our safe place.

"God is our refuge and strength, an ever-present help in trouble." (Psalm 46:1)

"How priceless is your unfailing love! Both high and low among men find refuge in the shadow of your wings." (Psalm 36:7)

"In the shelter of your presence you hide them from the intrigues of men; in your dwelling you keep them safe from accusing tongues." (Psalm 31:20)

These verses are good to memorize so that we can quickly be reminded of God's help when we don't feel emotionally or physically safe.

Whenever I've turned to the Lord for a quiet place, he has quieted my soul and filled the empty, longing places of my heart. This was true two years ago. During the morning passing period, I was relieved when one of my high school students, Krista, came into my room. She had been missing the day before—after visiting a friend in the hospital—and I had been concerned about her. I gave her a hug and asked her what had happened. To my horror it wasn't good. Friends of the patient had told her they'd give her a ride home but instead took her to their home and raped her. I quickly found out that I was the first adult Krista had told—even before her parents—and became the one who reported the crime. She needed a place to cope and feel safe, so my room and I provided her sanctuary for a while. However, when I became wiped out from the meetings and counseling and paperwork, I found that God was my refuge—the place where I could prayerfully release the hurt and anger I was feeling for Krista. Happily, she has recovered well in the last two years. She even recently introduced me to her fiancé, calling me her "other mom."

Maybe you desperately need a sanctuary yourself. Perhaps your husband has been unfaithful or the police have knocked on your door because your child was found with drugs. Perhaps you have been betrayed and are wondering whom you can trust. Do you need a safe place? Run to God, the Healer whose heart went out to the widow whose only son had died, the One who said, "Don't cry," and healed the boy (Luke 7:11-15). Run to this Comforter who said, "Do not let your hearts be troubled. Trust in God; trust also in me" (John 14:1). Run to the Savior, who spread out his arms and died for us so that we would never be separated from our Father, our sanctuary. There you will find shelter.

Prayer Starter

Lord, you are my Refuge and Strength, my Very Present Help in time of need. Thank you for welcoming me, sheltering me, and holding me close when I am troubled by the world around me. May I also extend your sanctuary to others when they need a safe place too. In Jesus' name, amen.

Fitness Tip

If you must walk alone, keep a mental list of those safe havens along your route. I have several doors I could knock on if I needed help. A cell phone might be wise to carry as well.

Chapter 46

Dumping Ground

DAILY PRAYERWALK
Read Psalm 13.

PRAYERWALK FOCUS
"How long, O LORD? Will you forget me forever? How long will you hide your face from me?"—Psalm 13:1

Sometimes my prayers sound like a sad country song. *My friend is mad at me. Someone stole my lawnmower. Why haven't you healed* _____? I take all my complaints and unload them at God's feet.

While it may seem wrong to be preoccupied with a list of issues, where else should we go but to God when we're hurting, sad, or troubled? The writers of Scripture often did this. The psalms often express some kind of complaint to God. The book of Lamentations, probably written by the prophet Jeremiah, is solely devoted to laments—mournful poems—about the destruction of Jerusalem in 586 B.C. All of the prophetic books contain laments, and Job is full of moaning and groaning.

Psalm 13 models how we might approach God in prayer with our unhappiness. The typical lament will list the issues the writer[39] has with God, then offer a verse or two at the end that expresses that final trust in him, no matter what the earthly situation looks like.

We see honest prayer here, which should be an encouragement to us to go to God no matter how we feel. The author wrote:

> How long, O LORD? Will you forget me forever?
>> How long will you hide your face from me?
> How long must I wrestle with my thoughts
>> and every day have sorrow in my heart?
> How long will my enemy triumph over me?
> Look on me and answer, O LORD my God.
>> Give light to my eyes, or I will sleep in death;
> my enemy will say, "I have overcome him,"
>> and my foes will rejoice when I fall. (verses 1-4)

This writer was being pursued successfully by an enemy. He is tormented by his sorrowful thoughts, but he wasn't hearing from God either. He had gotten to the point where he thought death was simpler. Haven't many of us felt like that at times? I have. God certainly knows how we feel—we might as well express it to him. What better place to go than to the Lord when we're sad, worried, or overwhelmed?

As I've studied psalms of lament, I've noticed that they usually have a turn, a point where the writer changes from despair to hope. This is evident in the last two verses of Psalm 13: "*But* I trust in your unfailing love; my heart rejoices in your salvation. I will sing to the LORD, for he has been good to me" (verses 5-6, emphasis added). The word *but* reminds us that even though life is falling apart, we can turn to our changeless, faithful God, who is still there, still trustworthy, still caring for us despite our problems.

Sometimes as I'm listing my frustrations to God, I will stop and think, *But!* Then I remember to recount those times when God has been faithful—the happy events, the times when the bills were paid, the days my children proclaimed their faith in Christ. Doing this helps me turn from my current woe to a future hope.

I had a pity party when Craig forgot my birthday last year. It was one of those important ones, a milestone I'd figured he wouldn't forget. But he did, and I was grouchy for days, even taking my grumbles to prayer. Finally God reminded me, *But!* I then remembered and thanked God for how Craig never grumbles when I leave for days at a time to speak or attend conferences, how he loves to take our kids backpacking, and how he had gifted me with a lovely pearl ring *and* flowers on Valentine's Day just the month before my birthday. Those remembrances provided the turn in my prayer for me, and I was able to leave my complaint with God.

So if you're feeling down, remember that a huge chunk of the Bible contains honest prayers by complaining men. Then go put on your walking shoes and lay your complaints at God's feet.

PRAYER STARTER

Lord, thank you that you welcome me, even when I'm angry or unhappy. You patiently hear my cries, comfort me, and then take the problems on yourself. Prod me to walk—run!—to you when I don't feel holy enough to pray. Turn my sadness to joy, my laments to praise. In Jesus' name, amen.

FITNESS TIP

If your muscles and joints are complaining, are you remembering to stretch fully when you're done? Hold these stretches for at least twenty seconds each:

- Reach your arms up as high as you can above your head.
- Put your arm behind your head, and push your elbow down with your other hand, as though you're trying to push your arm down your back. Repeat with other arm.
- Stand on one foot, and with your hand push the suspended foot into your bottom. Repeat with other leg.
- Lift your leg onto a chair or countertop, and straighten it. Repeat with other leg.
- Put your extended arms onto a wall, and lean into the wall.
- On the floor put your legs in a V, and try to touch one ear to the same side's knee. Repeat with other side.
- Then put the heels of your feet together, and pull them toward you on the floor.

You should do at least five minutes of stretching. Be faithful to this, and you shouldn't have attendant aches and pains.

Chapter 47

Meditating on His Word

Read Joshua 1:1-18.

PRAYERWALK FOCUS
"Do not let this Book of the Law depart from your mouth; meditate on it day and night, so that you may be careful to do everything written in it. Then you will be prosperous and successful."—Joshua 1:8

Have you ever been to an art museum and stared at a painting you liked or wanted to understand better? After a while you begin to notice the nuances of the artist's work, and you may find yourself so engrossed that you've lost track of anything else around you. Your thoughts are so focused on that artwork that perhaps you even imagine yourself in it. When you walk away, somehow the painting has changed you—given you new understanding or joy.

Meditating on God's Word has the same effect. When we meditate on God's Word, instead of taking it apart, we take it in and make it a part of us. We focus exclusively on a passage or verse or even a couple of words so that we're praying it. Meditating isn't a quick read-and-pray-the-Bible experience. Meditating means reading over and over and over, so many times that we have memorized the passage. We go beyond *what it says* to think *about what it means in general* and *what it means for us personally*—until we know how we are to respond to it. When we meditate on it, the living Word changes us—our understanding of who God is, who we are, what our life means, what purpose God has for us, any number of things, really!

I compare meditation to swimming in a lake. You can sit by a lake, study it, even dip your toes in it, but you won't know what the lake is fully like until you dive in and swim around awhile—even open your eyes underwater to see what's under the surface. The refreshment from the Word comes when we've really pondered and wondered over it.

Psalm 1 says that a man who meditates on the law is "like a tree planted by streams of water, which yields its fruit in season and whose leaf does not wither. Whatever he does prospers" (verse 3). After Moses died, the Lord promised prosperity and success to Joshua if he meditated on the law day and night (Joshua 1:8). In fulfillment of God's forty-year-old promise, Joshua was to take the Israelites across the Jordan River to the Promised Land. The job was formidable, however, as the Jews' numbers were in the millions with women and children, and the land was not vacant. Many fearless, godless peoples on the other side of the river were ready to fight rather than move.

Three times in his directive to the new leader, God told Joshua to "be strong and courageous." Other than to cross the river, the only specific direction God gave him was not to let the law depart from his mouth, but to meditate on it day and night so that he would be careful to do everything in it. That's some unusual battle plan: Meditate on the law!

Perhaps, though, that's also the best battle strategy for our lives. Instead of using our reason and forming well-laid plans, we can meditate on God's Word, imagining what God means for us individually. Some might think it's a bit odd to use the imagination to meditate. However, Richard Foster writes that "just as we believe that God can take our reason (fallen as it is) and sanctify it and use it for his good purpose, so we believe he can sanctify the imagination and use it for his good purposes."[40] If we really believe that the Bible was written for us, this leap won't be difficult. We simply put ourselves into a place of empathy as we're thinking about a verse or passage. In this way we can find God speaking to us through his Word. When we do, we'll reach that *aha!* moment that takes us deeper in prayer, deeper in our relationship with the Living Word. Dietrich Bonhoeffer said that just as Mary pondered all those words in her heart when she learned she would bear the Son of God, so we can ponder in our prayers, waiting for God to reveal his special insight to us.[41]

Years ago I had to take the National Teacher's Examination in English before I could get my teaching certification in California. The test would include questions about classic pieces of literature—titles, authors' and characters' names, literature periods, and more. It had been more than seventeen years since I'd graduated from college, and although I studied continuously for two solid months for that exam, I was afraid I'd fail. A friend had taken it twice and failed both times— and she had taken more English classes than I had.

The week of the exam a friend stopped by and suggested that I meditate on Philippians 4:13: "I can do all things through Him who strengthens me" (NASB). As I thought and prayed about that verse, I dwelled for a time on each separate word. I tried to picture myself as God saw me: I imagined that he saw me as a woman who would be a good teacher and as a good student who would pass the test. Soon God's truth pierced through my fear. I became convinced that God had appointed me to take that test and that with his help I would do well. I took the exam that Saturday and, a few weeks later, learned I had passed with a good score. Until that point I had never been a very confident person, but meditating on that verse changed my life. I still believe that with God's help I can do anything he asks me to do.

Pick a verse today—maybe today's PrayerWalk Focus or another from the passage—and meditate on those words as you walk today. Swim around in them awhile and see what God says to you.

PRAYER STARTER

Lord, thank you for all of your promises to me today that are now sealed on my heart. You will give me every place where I will set my feet. No one will be able to stand against me when I have your Word within me. You promise that you will be with me wherever I go, never leaving me or forsaking me. I delight in your care for me. In Jesus' name, amen.

FITNESS TIP

If you're approaching your senior years, you may want to have your doctor give you a stress test to determine how your heart responds to exercise.

Chapter 48

Embracing Silence

PrayerWalk Focus
"Be still, and know that I am God."—Psalm 46:10

Craig and I had a long engagement. Officially it was nine months long, but unofficially it stretched over four years. We began dating the spring of our senior year in high school. After graduation that summer he asked me to marry him. I thought it was too soon to make such a commitment, but I agreed that we'd marry someday after college. We saw each other just about every weekend.

We married on a September Saturday and spent most of our honeymoon driving from the San Francisco Bay Area up the coast to Oregon. The first couple of days we enjoyed a vacation cottage on a high bluff overlooking the Mendocino coast. I know we walked the beaches a lot, but I don't recall much of the coming or going of the ocean foam or the call of the shore birds or the misty air. I do remember the warmth of my hand in his and the absolute ecstasy that we were finally husband and wife. The rest of the world right then didn't matter at all—we were focused completely on each other.

This kind of loving companionship is the best way I can describe silent or contemplative prayer. I don't remember the day or the circumstance when I found myself in this type of silent, adoring prayer, but I do remember feeling so much love for God and his love for me that I simply ran out of words. It seemed as though everything I had—my limbs, my eyes, my pores even—were being spent worshiping the Lord who had created me and died for me.

In my silent adoration I find true contentment and intimacy with my Savior. The work of prayer—seeing the needs in my community and remembering family and friends—is done. Yes, I'm still prayer-walking, but my sight has turned from outward to upward, overwhelmed by the knowledge that God *wants* to be with me.

In fact, he invites me, saying:

"Come, all you who are thirsty, come to the waters." (Isaiah 55:1)

"Come to me, all you who are weary and burdened, and I will give you rest." (Matthew 11:28)

Behind the invitation is God's perfect love—his desire to meet my needs, his anticipation to bless me abundantly, and his longing to fellowship with *me*. At times, after I've laid all my praise and requests at his feet, it's as though God says to me, *I will take care of all those needs—just "Be still, and know that I am God"* (Psalm 46:10).

Doesn't this kind of prayer sound wonderful? It is, but our hearts are often so busy with lists that we can't hear the invitation to "be still." If this is a desire of your heart, but you don't sense the readiness, you might do some self-examination first, as suggested by Tricia McCary Rhodes, who lays out a journey into contemplative prayer in *The Soul at Rest*.[42] Basically, this first step is asking yourself if you honestly want to obey God completely and belong to him fully.

The next step toward silent prayer is a sense of anticipation—when your heart is fully turned toward God in adoration without words. In the last stage God responds, returning his holy love. Others write that this ecstatic sense of God's love is not automatic, but I've found that God has not left me adoring him without his love given to me in return.

In silent prayer I truly feel I'm walking with him, sensing many of the same benefits that Brother Lawrence has written about in his classic book *The Practice of the Presence of God*.[43] I've been strengthened in hope—worries do not ruin my day or plague my outlook. I do not let the things of this earth control my joy-o-meter: It wells up from that presence living within me. I have a growing boldness to talk about my faith and to pray that others will know God as I do. I find that I don't have to mull over decisions much: His direction for my life is clear. Nor do I have to psyche myself up for worship; it's as natural now as breathing.

Jeanne Guyon wrote that eventually it's possible to experience oneness with God. "Self-effort gradually decreases. Eventually, it ceases altogether. When self-effort ceases, your will is passive before God.... This is union. Divine union. The self is ended. The human will is totally passive and responds to every movement of God's will."[44]

This is what I want—to be one with my Lord in heart, head, and purpose.

This is also what I wish for you—that as you faithfully pray, day after day, you will experience the intimate friendship of our Lord who invites you to "be still" with him.

PRAYER STARTER

Lord, thank you that you invite me to be still with you. It amazes me that you seek my company and share so freely your love for me. I pray that I'll grow so much in my love for you that I cannot contain it anymore so that it spills over and over to others and to you. In Jesus' name, amen.

FITNESS TIP

WalkSport America sponsors a national mall-walking program, which has swipe cards for use in member malls around the country. For more information call 800-757-9255 or visit www.walksport.com.[45]

Chapter 49

First Impulse

DAILY PRAYERWALK
Read James 5:13-20.

PRAYERWALK FOCUS
"The prayer of a righteous man is powerful and effective."
—James 5:16

A few years ago I received a good lesson in regard to both self-control and prayer. A friend, Mary, called me up with several prayer requests. Her life was falling down all around her—rebellious son, unfaithful husband, job misery, and church failure. With each request, I spilled out my I-Ts—"I think…," and I had at least several for each of her problems.

Finally she said, "Janet, if I wanted your opinion about what to do, I would have asked you. What I wanted was for you to listen and to pray for me."

She was absolutely right. In my usual tendency to control or fix the situation, I had tried to provide solutions to her problems rather than empathy and prayer. I prayed for her right then, thankful for a hard but good lesson in friendship.

James teaches that prayer should be our first impulse when he writes: "Is any one of you in trouble? He should pray. Is anyone happy? Let him sing songs of praise. Is any one of you sick? He should call the elders of the church to pray over him" (James 5:13-14). When the washing machine clunks and stops…for good…I should pray. When I find my car door smashed in a shopping center parking lot with no note on the windshield, I should pray. When my printer decides to die in the middle of a deadline, I should pray. God knew each of these events would happen before they did, and he has allowed them. He cares more about my response than about the event.

I didn't always believe that I should pray for the ups and downs and little things of my day. I thought I'd just be bogging the Lord down with too much prayer trivia. But one day I was shopping with my friend Hannah, and she even prayed for things like groceries! At first I thought that a bit weird, but by the end of the day, I noticed that she was doing a whole lot better at her shopping dollar-wise than I was. The next shopping trip I asked God to help me do efficient school shopping for Bethany. I ended up spending half the amount in half the time I had planned. Not only did I stay under budget, but I went home in a better mood too.

Since then I've learned that praying for my day helps me pray in response to whatever happens throughout the day. If I pray before I teach a class, and it goes well, I thank God. If the students are rude or complaining, there's a greater likelihood that I'll pray for them than get angry or resentful. When prayer is my first response, it shows that my heart was first tuned to God rather than my own agenda and that I rely more on him than on the things that could otherwise control my life.

When our initial response is prayer, we've put God in the center of our daily activities. We're telling him, "I trust you for this."

PRAYER STARTER

Train me, Lord, to turn to you first in all of the ups and downs of my day. Help me put my eyes on you as I begin my day so that my reactions are a prayerful seeking rather than a knee-jerk reacting. May I praise you with each good thing and take you my questions when I wonder. In Jesus' name, amen.

FITNESS TIP

Walking for Health recommends that if you get a stabbing pain in your side while you're walking, stop walking. Then use three fingers to "press on the area where the pain is greatest until it stops hurting. Or gently massage the area." Work up slowly to your desired walking pace to avoid those cramps.[46]

Chapter 50

Praying Without Ceasing

DAILY PRAYERWALK
Read 1 Thessalonians 5:1-18.

PRAYERWALK FOCUS
"Pray without ceasing."—1 Thessalonians 5:17, NASB

With each new day that I spend prayerwalking and reading God's Word, I have a sense that I am in training. I'm learning how to see the world as God would—filled with needs. Because my focus is becoming more outward, I'm beginning to get a vision of what Paul meant when he said we should "pray without ceasing" (1 Thessalonians 5:17, NASB).

The best way I can explain how you can pray all day long is to take you through one of my teaching days. Come walk with me, friend...

My friend June meets me on Friday at 5 A.M. at my house, and we immediately head down Main Street. The stars are so bright in our dark mountain sky that I fall easily into silent praise of the Creator who would gift us with such a delightful dot-to-dot decoration for insomniacs or us early risers. *You delight me, God.*

June and I have an understanding. Sometimes we pray silently.

Sometimes we pray together. And if we chat, we know the listener is praying for the other's needs. This morning she shares about her concerns for her son and grandson who might face overseas military duty, and I pray for their protection and reconciliation with God. When she talks of her worry over her older model car, I pray that God would lead her to just the right replacement. As she speaks of her desire to finish a book proposal, I ask God to give her wisdom and determination to finish it. *Thank you for friends, God.*

Together we pray for the businesses that line Main Street and all of the owners by name. When a car passes us with its bright lights on, that reminds me to pray for those commuting long distances to work, especially that the migrating deer would stay out of their paths. As we near my husband's hayfields, I pray for rain after our year of drought and that he can get his bale wagon fixed sooner so the hay can be picked up out of the fields before the wet season starts. *Help him, Lord.*

For the first couple of laps up and down the street, I keep coughing. It's annoying until I realize that the smoky air is probably from the forest fire down the canyon. And that reminds me to pray for the firefighters' safety and for those whose homes might also be threatened by the fire. Now tuned into the smells around me, I take in the sweetness of the steam coming from the lumber mill's power plant. It's still running, despite the mill's closing earlier this year, and I thank God for that fact, as well as for the jobs that dozens of others have found after working at the mill for many years. *You are our faithful Provider.*

After an hour-plus of wonderful prayer, the rest of the day almost rushes past me, but God keeps bringing me back to a prayerful focus. When I find my paintings at a tilt, I brush away annoyance, straighten them out, and praise God for my playful children. When I notice the dog hair dancing on the edges of the kitchen floor, I thank God for the newest addition to our home, our border collie, Patsy. When Bethany moans in her sleep, I step into her room, put my hand on her head, and ask God to calm her spirit and bless her day. When the newspaper still hasn't come at seven o'clock, I pray for my high school student and his family who drive a combined total of three hundred miles before dawn each day to deliver papers in our rural area. *Be their Protector, God.*

I step into a prayer-run of sorts as I wake our two youngest kids, feed them breakfast, and whoosh to school in my ninety-second commute. I ask God to bless the boys who hang out in the Bear Cave, a bench-lined corner of our school behind my room. They're mostly younger boys, awkward and physical as they relate to each other. I've had to train my whole countenance over the last few years to greet them warmly, and they "hello" me back. *Live in me, Lord.*

I think I'm going to slide slowly into the day, with a first period preparation, but the teacher who uses my classroom during that time is called away to mother her stomach-sick boy, and I'm the instant sub for chatty freshmen in world geography. Again I'm training myself to turn from inner complaints ("I need this prep time, God!") to prayer—for the teacher and her son, for the students whose names I don't even know, for peace across the world as they're coloring continents on their butcher-paper maps. *And let it begin with me in this classroom.*

I pray for my juniors up and down rows of the next two classes. I pray for Todd, who's been absent all week. As I hand out grade updates, I pray over those failing. *Help them do their work, Lord. Help them as they cope in less-than-perfect homes.* The prayers are changing me. I find myself extending grace on missed assignments: "Ask your PE teacher if you can come make up that essay next period." "I'll help you sign up for the SAT II on my credit card, and your mom can pay me back." "I'm going to let you folks redo those first couple of vocabulary tests." *Thanks for the cool day, God.*

After school I'm ready to collapse, but my kids and I go by the elementary school to help close up the book fair in its last moments of a three-day run. It's been a week like that for me, with several doctor appointments, lessons, and book events filling my after-school hours and evenings. I'm leaning toward self-pity, but then I see the moms packing up the hundreds of books... I pray for those who volunteer their days to help teachers and aides and librarians and more. *Thank you, God, for all the hands that work together to teach our children.*

As I fix dinner, I pray over newspaper headlines. As Bethany practices piano, I rejoice that God has given us sound that comes together as music—and that both my daughters have the gift to delight. As I read the Bible and a book about marriage, I ask God to speak to my heart and make me more like Jesus. And then I go to bed and sleep for—can you believe it?—TWELVE hours. I guess my week of prayer had finally caught up with me. *Good night, Father.*

I bet you can find that you can pray without ceasing today. Join me as I take off the blinders of my daily planner and see what God would have me notice. And in the process, I bet we find that we're right in the middle of his joy all day long. Thanks for walking with me, friend. Now go with God on your own prayerwalk—and may he bless you greatly and answer your prayers.

PRAYER STARTER

Thank you, Father, for the suggestion in your Word that we can pray without ceasing. Develop within me your eyesight for others—giving thanks for them and praying for their needs. And in the process may I find that your unconditional love is spilling over into my prayers and the way I relate to others and that joy has replaced the dread, boredom, and indifference of my soul. In Jesus' name, amen.

FITNESS TIP

For cold or changeable weather, dress in layers. The layer next to your skin should be of a wicking fabric that moves moisture away from your skin. Fleece works well for a middle layer. The outer layer should be wind and water resistant. (Gore-Tex and similar materials will allow sweat to evaporate without letting rain in.)

Notes

1. I've even written a book about this subject: *Girlfriend Gatherings: Creative Ways to Stay Connected* (Eugene, Oreg.: Harvest House, 2001).

2. Those interested in the various names for God may want to read one or more of the following books, all published by Moody Press of Chicago: *Names of God* by Nathan Stone (1944), *Names of Christ* by T. C. Horton and Charles E. Hurlburt (1994), and *Names of the Holy Spirit* by Ray Pritchard (1995).

3. Adapted from Psalm 8:1,3 and Philippians 2:10-11.

4. Mark Fenton and Seth Bauer, *The 90-Day Fitness Walking Program* (New York: Perigee, 1995).

5. Casey Meyers, *Walking: A Complete Guide to the Complete Exercise* (New York: Random House, 1992), 84.

6. Dag Hammarskjöld, *Markings*, trans. Leif Sjoberg and W. H. Auden (New York: Knopf, 1966), 124.

7. D. Guthrie, and others, *The New Bible Commentary Revised* (Grand Rapids: Eerdmans, 1970), 824.

8. Meyers, *Walking*, 225.

9. Adapted from Psalm 119:9-16.

10. Shirley Pope Waite, "Standing in the Gap," *NIV Women's Devotional Bible* (Grand Rapids: Zondervan, 1995), 924.

11. T. L. Marshall, "Prodigal," *Decision* 42, no. 6 (June 2001): 31.

12. W. E. Vine, *An Expository Dictionary of New Testament Words* (Old Tappan, N.J.: Revell, 1966), 172.

13. Lucinda Secrest McDowell, *Amazed by Grace* (Nashville: Broadman & Holman, 1996), 4.

14. Mark Fenton and Margit Feury, "Make Your Walk a Workout," *Walking* 15, no. 4 (June 2000): 55.

15. The address and phone are American Tract Society, Box 462008, Garland, TX 75046-2008; 1-800-548-7228.

16. Meyers, *Walking*, 117.

17. Mark Bricklin and Maggie Spilner, eds., *Prevention's Practical Encyclopedia of Walking for Health* (Emmaus, Pa.: Rodale Press, 1992), 129-30.

18. Henry T. Blackaby and Claude V. King, *Experiencing God: Knowing and Doing the Will of God* (Nashville: LifeWay Press, 1990), 83, 87, 95, 105.

19. Blackaby and King, *Experiencing God*, 79.

20. If the idea of God's speaking to you personally sounds strange, could it be that, like Samuel, you don't yet know him? Have you established a relationship with him by inviting Jesus Christ into your heart? By uttering this prayer you can begin that line of communication: "Lord, I acknowledge that I need you in my life. I ask you to forgive me of my sins and to live within my heart and soul forever. In Jesus' name. Amen." If you prayed this prayer, I rejoice with you and encourage you to get to know God's voice by reading his Word, praying, and worshiping with other believers.

21. Anne Kashiwa and James Rippe, M.D., *Fitness Walking for Women* (New York: Perigee, 1987).

22. Stephanie Oakes, "Women and Workouts," *USA Weekend*, 28 September 2001, 14.

23. Phrases from the following verses in Psalms are echoed in the Jonah 2:2-9 passage: 11:4; 18:5-6; 30:3; 42:6-7; 50:14; 61:8; 62:1; 65:1; 66:13; 69:1-2; 86:13; 12:1. There may be others as well.

24. Mark Fenton, *The Complete Guide to Walking* (Guilford, Conn.: Lyons Press, 2001), 129.

25. David's story is told in 1 Samuel 15–31 and all of 2 Samuel.

26. Fenton, *The Complete Guide to Walking*, 145.

27. Liz Neporent, *Fitness Walking for Dummies* (Foster City, Calif.: IDG Books, 2000), 269.

28. We hear a lot about the word *call* in church. A call is simply God's election or commission of you or me for a special purpose. He may call us to perform a unique function, job, or ministry for him. God makes that call clear through prayer that is confirmed by his Word and perhaps also through others' encouragement and circumstances.

29. John Maxwell, *Partners in Prayer* (Nashville: Nelson, 1996), 78-9.

30. Herbert Lockyer, *All the Prayers of the Bible* (Grand Rapids: Zondervan, 1959), 272.

31. Fenton and Bauer, *The 90-Day Fitness Walking Program,* 98-9.

32. Elmer L. Towns, *Fasting for Spiritual Breakthrough: A Guide to Nine Biblical Fasts* (Ventura, Calif.: Regal, 1996), 17.

33. Richard J. Foster, *Celebration of Discipline* (New York: Harper, 1988), 54.

34. Dallas Willard, *The Spirit of the Disciplines: Understanding How God Changes Lives* (New York: Harper & Row, 1988), 166.

35. Bill Bright, *Seven Basic Steps to Successful Fasting and Prayer* (Orlando: New Life Publications, 1995), 7-16.

36. Richard J. Foster, *Prayer: Finding the Heart's True Home* (New York: HarperSanFrancisco, 1992), 229, 234.

37. Neporent, *Fitness Walking for Dummies,* 80-1.

38. Zerubbabel's name means "born or begotten in Babylon." He is referred to in historical accounts as Sheshbazzar.

39. This psalm is attributed to David, but many of the psalms that are labeled as "A psalm of David" could have been written about him rather than by him.

40. Foster, *Prayer,* 148.

41. Dietrich Bonhoeffer, *The Way to Freedom* (New York: Harper & Row), 59, quoted in Foster, *Prayer,* 146.

42. Tricia McCary Rhodes, *The Soul at Rest: A Journey into Contemplative Prayer* (Minneapolis: Bethany, 1996), 198-9.

43. Brother Lawrence, *The Practice of the Presence of God* (North Brunswick, N.J.: Bridge-Logos, 1999), 134-6.

44. Jeanne Guyon, *Experiencing the Depths of Jesus Christ* (Sargent, Ga.: SeedSowers, 1975), 133.

45. Fenton, *The Complete Guide to Walking*, 247.

46. Mark Bricklin, ed., *Walking for Health* (Emmaus, Pa.: Rodale Press, 1992), 73.

For information about Janet Holm McHenry's speaking availability,
you may contact her at:
P.O. Box 750
Loyalton, CA 96118
or through her Web sites:
www.janetmchenry.com
and
www.dailyprayerwalking.com

To learn more about WaterBrook Press and view
our catalog of products, log on to our Web site:
www.waterbrookpress.com

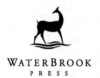

WATERBROOK
PRESS